Ester De Giuli Angelo Sala

ENGLISH FOR PHARMACY

Biotechnologies, Drugs, Natural Remedies and Cosmetics

EDITORE ULRICO HOEPLI MILANO

via Hoepli 5, 20121 Milano (Italy)
tel. +39 02 864871 – fax +39 02 8052886
e-mail hoepli@hoepli.it

www.hoepli.it

ISBN 978-88-203-4475-7

Ristampa:

4 2025

Realizzazione editoriale: Thèsis Contents S.r.l., Firenze-Milano

Copertina: mncg S.r.l., Milano

Stampa: Legodigit S.r.l., Lavis (Trento)

Printed in Italy

CONTENTS

Unit 10 Scientific Papers

Unit 11 Introduction to Chemistry

Unit 12 Natural Remedies

Unit 13 Herbal Drugs

PRESENTAZIONE

La lingua inglese è divenuta lo strumento base per la comunicazione in campo scientifico e non solo. A fronte dell'obbligatorietà di questa competenza, il professionista del farmaco si trova di fronte a due difficoltà: da un lato, una conoscenza della lingua scolastica, quasi sempre indirizzata in senso letterario o comunque con riferimenti scientifici molto modesti; dall'altro, una pratica dell'inglese parlato troppo spesso non sufficiente e che rende molto difficile comprendere vocaboli scientifici pronunciati a volte in modo inatteso.

Come Preside della Facoltà di Farmacia ho visto con grande soddisfazione l'impegno della prof.ssa De Giuli nel trasmettere agli studenti alcune conoscenze fondamentali per poter utilizzare lo strumento dell'inglese scientifico. In primo luogo è necessario conoscere i temi principali dell'inglese impiegato in farmaceutica, in secondo luogo è importante sapere applicare una lingua non propria a obiettivi ben precisi e rilevanti per la professione che si è scelta. Fra questi diversi sono quelli svolti nel testo, che trovo particolarmente apprezzabile e che allarga le cognizioni linguistiche, introducendo infatti argomenti come le sperimentazioni cliniche, l'industria farmaceutica, la farmacovigilanza e tutta una serie di temi che comprendono anche naturalmente le cosiddette *application*, con la stesura di CV e le linee generali della redazione di un testo da presentare a una rivista scientifica o a un congresso. Quest'ultimo è un argomento spesso doloroso. I *referees* degli articoli di autori italiani tendono spesso a sottolineare che il testo richiede una "revision by an English speaking person"! Può essere che l'utilizzo di questo volume non modifichi in modo sostanziale il destino di molti manoscritti che cadono sotto questo capestro forse un po' snobistico. Tuttavia è caro per me apprezzare come i due Autori, Angelo Sala, brillante docente con un prestigioso curriculum statunitense, ed Ester De Giuli, entrambi della Facoltà che ho l'onore di presiedere, abbiano deciso di affrontare questa problematica, fornendo uno strumento del quale certamente si sentiva la necessità.

Il gap finanziario, tecnologico e culturale con i Paesi anglosassoni non è certamente dovuto solo alla lingua, ma la miglior percezione dello strumento linguistico, la potenzialità di interagire meglio con il mondo del lavoro e con il mondo scientifico rimane una priorità. Sono certo che l'intento di questo libro risponda a tale esigenza e non posso che augurarmi che abbia ampia diffusione.

CESARE SIRTORI
Ordinario di Farmacologia Clinica
Preside della Facoltà di Farmacia
Università degli Studi di Milano

INTRODUZIONE

To Edoardo, Francesca, Maria Nicole and Valeria,
future citizens of the world

English for Pharmacy è stato concepito principalmente per l'utilizzo da parte degli studenti dei Corsi di laurea della Facoltà di indirizzo farmaceutico, quali Farmacia, Chimica e Tecnologie Farmaceutiche, Tecniche Erboristiche, Tossicologia dell'Ambiente, Biotecnologie Farmaceutiche, ma può rappresentare un ausilio pratico anche per tutti gli operatori del settore che devono acquisire dimestichezza con la lingua inglese applicata all'ambito farmaceutico.
Il testo procede muovendo da una conoscenza di base della lingua, proponendo materiali testuali autentici attinti dal mondo accademico, dalle aziende del settore, dalle riviste specializzate, dagli enti governativi, nella consapevolezza che i linguaggi specialistici vanno acquisiti "sul campo" con l'obiettivo di soddisfare le esigenze linguistiche insieme agli obiettivi informativi.
L'apparato didattico mira all'acquisizione del linguaggio specialistico, allo sviluppo delle abilità di comprensione e di produzione scritta. Ogni capitolo presenta la stessa struttura: l'argomento principale viene sviluppato attraverso diversi testi cui fanno seguito note, approfondimenti e numerosi esercizi che mirano a facilitare l'acquisizione del vocabolario specialistico, a implementare le abilità di comprensione e le capacità di produzione scritta, insieme alle informazioni utili sugli aspetti della cultura anglo-sassone riferiti all'ambito professionale/farmaceutico.
Un'appendice di schede grammaticali completa il volume, fornendo il supporto a fronte di eventuali incertezze. Per dare agli utilizzatori la possibilità di meglio familiarizzarsi con la pronuncia anglosassone il volume è corredato di file audio in formato Mp3 con la lettura dei brani principali.
Il volume si presenta come uno strumento articolato, aggiornato e pratico, all'interno del quale ogni docente può costruire il proprio itinerario didattico.

Le chiavi degli esercizi proposti nel volume sono consultabili on-line all'indirizzo www.hoeplieditore.it/4475-7 dove è anche possibile scaricare i file Audio.

UNIT 1

CLINICAL TRIALS: TESTING MEDICAL PRODUCTS IN PEOPLE

WHAT ARE CLINICAL TRIALS?

Clinical trials, also known as clinical studies, test potential treatments in human volunteers to see whether they should be approved for wider use in the general population. A treatment could be a drug, medical device, or biologic, such as a vaccine, blood product, or gene therapy. Potential treatments, however, must be studied in laboratory animals first to determine potential toxicity before they can be tried in people. Treatments having acceptable safety profiles and showing the most promise are then moved into clinical trials.

Although "new" may imply "better", it is not known whether the potential medical treatment offers benefit to patients until clinical research on the treatment is complete. Clinical trials are an integral part of new product discovery and development and are required before a new product can be brought to the market.

Every clinical trial is carefully designed to answer certain research questions. A trial plan called protocol maps out what study procedures will be done, by whom, and why. Products are often tested to see how they compare to standard treatments or to no treatment.

Clinical trial teams include doctors and nurses, as well as other health care professionals. These teams check the health of participants at the beginning of the trial and assess whether those persons are eligible to participate. Those found eligible – and who agree to participate – are given specific instructions, and then monitored and carefully assessed during the trial and after it is completed.

Done at hospitals and research centers, clinical trials are conducted in phases.

Phase 1 trials, primarily concerned with safety, try to determine dosing, document how a drug is metabolized and excreted, and identify acute side effects. This phase usually only involves small numbers of participants (between 20 and 80), and are usually undertaken in healthy volunteers. Increasing doses of the drugs are administrated during the studies, and blood samples collected.

Phase 2 trials include more participants (usually 100-300) who have the disease or condition that the product potentially could treat. In Phase 2 trials, researchers seek to gather further safety data and preliminary evidence of the drug's efficacy, and they develop and refine research methods for future trials. If the Phase 2 trials indicate that the drug may be effective and the risks are considered acceptable, given the observed efficacy and the severity of the disease, the drug moves to Phase 3.

In **Phase 3 trials**, the drug is studied in a larger number of people with the disease (approximately 1,000-3,000 but up to 20,000). This phase further tests the product's effectiveness, monitors side effects and, in some cases, compares new treatments with the existing one to demonstrate long term safety and tolerance. As more and more participants are tested over longer periods of time, the less common side effects are more likely to be revealed.

Phase 4 trials are generally performed after a product is already approved on the market to find out more about the treatment's long-term risks, benefits, and optimal use, or to test the product in different populations of people, such as children or elderly.

Phase 2 and Phase 3 clinical trials generally involve a "standard procedure of control". In many studies one group of volunteers is given a "test" drug or treatment (test group) while the other group (control group) is given either a standard treatment for the illness or an inactive substance that has no treatment value (placebo).

The treatments that trial participants receive are often decided by a process called randomization. This process can be compared to a coin toss that is done by computer. During clinical trials randomization assures that treatment selection will be free of any bias.

In conjunction with randomization, a feature known as blinding helps ensure that bias doesn't affect the trial or the interpretation of its results. Single-blinding means participants do not know whether they are receiving the experimental drug or a placebo. A double-blinded trial means that neither the research team nor the participants know who is receiving the experimental drug. The keys that allow the identification of the treatment used are made available only at the end of the study.

[A special report from *FDA Consumer Magazine*, adapted from]

Informed consent is a process that includes:

- information about the possible risks and benefits of a treatment;
- information about the risks and benefits of other options, including not getting treatment;
- answering to possible questions and requests of additional information by the patient;
- time (if needed) to discuss the plan with family or advisors;
- communication of the decision to the doctor or treatment team, eventually through the use of specifically designed forms (in case of written consent).

All medical care requires the consent of the patient (or someone who is authorized to consent for the patient) before the care plan is carried out.

Your signature on the form is taken to be evidence that this took place. If you decide that you do not want the procedure or treatment, you would not sign the consent form.

Exercise 1

Decide which statements are true (T) or false (F).

	T	F
1. Clinical trials are required before a new drug is on sale.		
2. Phase 1 trials generally involve healthy volunteers.		
3. Drug trials with human subjects are carried out after tests on laboratory animals.		
4. Once accepted into a study, clinical trial participants should be randomly assigned to treatments.		
5. In single blind studies patients do not know whether they are in the treatment or not.		
6. A double blind study is when the test is carried out with only two patients.		
7. Phase 3 is basically about long-term risks.		

8. Phase 4 trials are generally carried out on drugs which have been refused by the market ■ ■
9. The "standard procedure of control" is generally carried out in phases 2 and 3. ■ ■
10. Blind trials are helpful in trying not to affect the interpretation of results. ■ ■

Exercise 2

Fill in the blanks with the words from the box.

• designed • drug • health • involves • treat • long-term • randomization • researchers • tolerance • treatment • participants • concerned • determine • disease • effectiveness • risks • research • develop • side • effective • trial

1. Every clinical trial is carefully .... to answer certain .... questions.
2. These teams check the .... of participants at the beginning of the ....
3. Phase 1 trials, primarily .... with safety, try to .... dosing and document how a .... is metabolized.
4. This phase usually only .... small numbers of participants.
5. This trial includes participants who have the .... or condition that the product potentially could ....
6. They .... and research methods for future trials.
7. This indicates that the drug may be .... and the .... are considered acceptable.
8. Phase 3 tests the product's .... and monitors .... effects.
9. .... compare new treatments with the existing one to demonstrate .... safety and ....
10. The .... that trial .... receive is often decided by a process called ....

WORD FILE

- **Bias:** a tendency to be in favour or against something, prejudice. *On the bias:* diagonally. *Bias:* diagonal. *To bias:* to cause to form fixed opinions without enough information to judge.
- **Blind:** not able to see. *The blind:* i ciechi. *Blind:* tendina a rullo.
- **Device:** a piece of equipment intended for a particular purpose.
- **Disease:** illness or unhealthy condition caused by infection, a disorder etc. but not by accident.
- **Drug:** something (a medicine) that makes you better when you are ill. Something that people eat, smoke or inject because it makes them feel excited or happy. *Over-the-counter drugs:* drugs which can be obtained without prescription from a doctor.
- **Effective:** producing the desired result (efficace). **Pay attention** *Effettivo:* real, actual.
- **Health:** the state of being well in the body and mind, and free from disease.

- **Healthy:** sano.
- **Illness:** unhealthy state of the body or mind, disease.
- **Placebo:** a preparation, which has no pharmacologic effect, given for psychological effect, or as a control in evaluating a drug.
- **Random:** without any plan, aim or pattern. *At random:* a caso.
- **Safety:** the condition of being safe, free from harm, danger or risk. *Safe:* sicuro, salvo, certo.
- **Side effect:** an effect, often one that is unexpected or unwanted, happening in addition to the one that is intended.
- **Trial:** the act of testing to ensure quality, but also: investigation of a case before a judge (processo).
- **Volunteer (to):** to offer one's services or help without payment or reward. *Volunteer:* a person who volunteers to do a job.

- **Agree to (to):** essere d'accordo con. *Agreement:* accordo. *As far as I'm concerned:* per quanto mi riguarda.
- **Assess (to):** valutare, stimare.
- **By chance:** per caso.
- **Carry (to):** trasportare. *Carrier:* vettore.
- **Carry out (to):** effettuare, compiere.
- **Choice:** scelta.
- **Concerned with:** trattare, riguardare. *To be concerned about something:* essere preoccupati per. *To be concerned for somebody.*
- **Further:** ulteriore.
- **Gather (to):** raccogliere.
- **Professional:** professionale (a.), professionista (n.).

Pay attention

If, whether ➢ se

I don't know whether he is right.
I don't know if he is right.
Ask him if it's late.
Ask him whether it's late.

Whether ➢ quando si tratta di una scelta o di un dubbio fra due alternative
I don't know whether he likes it or not.

If ➢ quando introduce una condizione
If he doesn't come I'll leave.
If you agree say yes.

Exercise 3

Fill in the gaps with a suitable word from the passage.

1. Every clinical trial is carefully .... to answer certain .... questions.
2. Potential treatments must be studied in .... first to determine potential ....
3. Phase 1 usually .... small numbers of ....

4. The treatments that trial participants .... is often decided by a process called ....

5. As more and .... participants are tested over longer .... of time, the less common .... are more likely to be revealed.
6. In conjunction with ...., a feature known as blinding helps ensure that .... doesn't affect the trial or the interpretation of its results.

PLACEBOS

Placebos are substances that are made to resemble drugs but do not contain an active compound. A placebo is made to look exactly like a real drug but is made of an inactive substance such as starch or sugar.
Placebos are usually used in research studies. Placebos can result in or be coincidentally associated with many changes, both desiderable and undesiderable. This phenomenon, called the "placebo effect", appears to have two components: anticipation of results, usually optimistic, from taking a drug (sometimes called suggestibility) and spontaneous change. Sometimes people improve spontaneously, without treatment. If spontaneous change – whether positive or negative – occurs after a placebo is taken, the placebo may incorrectly be credited or blamed for the result.
Some people seem more susceptible to the placebo effect than others. People who have a positive opinion of drugs, doctors, nurses and hospitals are more likely to respond favourably to placebos than are people who have a negative opinion. Some people who are particularly susceptible to placebos tend to become compulsive about using the drug; they tend to increase the dose, and they develop withdrawal symptoms when they are deprived of the placebo.

Exercise 4

Translate the fragments in italics into English.

1. A placebo is made *per apparire esattamente come un farmaco reale* but do not contain any active drug.

   ....

2. This phenomenon, *chiamato effetto placebo*, appears to have two components.

   ....

3. People who have *un'opinione positiva dei farmaci*, doctors, nurses and hospitals *sono più probabili* to respond favourably to placebos than are *persone che hanno un'opinione negativa*.

   ....

4. They tend *ad aumentare la dose e sviluppano* withdrowal symptoms *quando privati del placebo*.

   ....

Exercise 5

Here are six definitions. Match them with words (nouns, verbs or others) in the passage.

1. A white tasteless substance forming an important part of foods such as grain, rice, potatoes and beans.

   ....

2. Very difficult to stop or control.

   ....

3. The complex of physical and psychological disturbance observed in addicts when they stop taking the addicting agent.

   ....

4. To consider someone or something responsible for something bad.

   ....

5. A sweet white or brown substance which is obtained from plants and used in food and drinks.

   ....

6. An outward or noticeable sign of disease.

   ....

Exercise 6

Read this media release and tick true (T) or false (F).

Basel, June 17, 20.. – Novartis today announced details of two new long-term outcome studies in its landmark ASPIRE HIGHER clinical trial program which has expanded to involve more than 35,000 patients in 14 trials. The series of trials that comprise ASPIRE HIGHER now form the largest and most far-reaching cardio-renal outcomes program worldwide.

The newly-launched studies will evaluate the organ protection potential of the first-in-class direct renin inhibitor Rasilez, known as Tekturna® in the US, for the treatment of heart failure and prevention of cardiovascular disease in the elderly, a patient segment that is predicted to more than double between 2000 and 2030.

A third megatrial already under way is studying cardio-renal outcomes in diabetes.

High blood pressure is a sign that many organs in the body could be under threat. Rasilez/Tekturna works by directly inhibiting renin, an enzyme that triggers a process leading to high blood pressure and organ damage. By inhibiting renin at the point of activation, Rasilez/Tekturna provides effective blood pressure reductions and may also afford greater protection against complications such as organ damage.

One quarter of the world's population, or approximately one billion people, are now affected by high blood pressure. This figure is projected to rise to 1.56 billion by 2025, a 60% increase over the current figure. In the US alone, the direct and indirect costs of high blood pressure in 2008 are estimated at USD 69.4 billion.

The ASPIRE HIGHER clinical program includes three major outcome studies:

- ALTITUDE will determine whether Rasilez/Tekturna, added to conventional therapy, delays heart and kidney complications in around 8,600 patients with type 2 diabetes at high risk for cardiovascular and renal events. The study began in late 2007 with completion anticipated by 2012.

- ATMOSPHERE will evaluate the effects of Rasilez/Tekturna on cardiovascular morbidity and mortality in patients with acute and chronic congestive heart failure on top of standard therapy.
- APOLLO will assess the effectiveness of Rasilez/Tekturna in preventing cardiovascular morbidity and mortality in elderly patients with or without high blood pressure and other risk factors.

		T	F
1.	Aspire Higher is a landmark concerning clinical trials carried out by Novartis.	▪	▪
2.	The two drugs called Rasilez and Tekturna have slightly different components.	▪	▪
3.	There are predictions for a raise in cardiovascular diseases in elderly patients in the future years.	▪	▪
4.	Rasilez treatments can assure blood pressure reductions.	▪	▪
5.	Novartis is carrying out four trials in the field of cardio-renal diseases.	▪	▪
6.	High blood pressure affects a large part of the world population but a decrease in the number of patients is expected in future years.	▪	▪
7.	One of the trials is supposed to evaluate whether Tekturna can improve life to patients with type 2 diabetes who are at risk.	▪	▪
8.	Another trial will assess the effectiveness of Rasilez in elderly population with risk factors.	▪	▪

Exercise 7

Read the passage and answer the questions.

Why participate in a Clinical Trial?

People volunteer to participate in clinical trials for different reasons. Some volunteer because they want to help advance medical knowledge. Others have tried all available treatments for their condition without success. In a 2000 Harris Poll of cancer clinical trial participants, 76 percent of the respondents said they participated because they believed that the trial offered the best quality of care for their disease. Helping other people and receiving more and better attention for their own specific disease were other reasons cited.

People should not, however, be tempted to enroll in a clinical trial simply because a potential treatment is being offered free during a study, or because of the promise of money, says David Banks, an FDA pharmacist.

People attracted by compensation may overlook the known risks, or they may fail to adequately appreciate the potential for discovery of serious new side effects during clinical testing of a new treatment. Clinical trials are generally not a means for patients to receive long-term treatment for their chronic disease still clinical trials often represent an option to be seriously taken into consideration.

What are the risks? Some treatments being studied can have unpleasant, or even serious, side effects. Often these are temporary and end when the treatment is stopped. Others, however, can be permanent. Some side effects appear during treatment, and others may not show up until after the study is over. The risks depend on the treatment being studied and the health of the people participating in the trial. All known risks must be fully explained by the researchers before the trial begins. If new risk information becomes available during the trial, participants must be informed.

[A Special Report from *FDA Consumer Magazine*]

1. Do people take part in clinical trials only for the love of scientific progress? Explain the different reasons.

....

....

....

2. Why can people fail to consider the risks of side effects during a clinical trial?

....

....

....

3. Which kind of risks can volunteers have?

....

....

....

4. What are the duties of researchers towards participants?

....

....

....

Exercise 8

Read this new passage about clinical trials and fill in the blanks with the words from the box. (Pay attention! The given words are more than what you need.)

• safely • diseases • volunteer • whether • health authorities • side effects
• testing • for sale • phases • market • safety • effectiveness • larger • small
• potentially • drug • patients • treatments • health • lungs • efficacy

Clinical trials are research studies which try to answer scientific questions and find better ways to treat or prevent .... A clinical trial is conducted to determine .... a new drug or treatment is both safe and effective in people. These research studies rely on patients who volunteer to participate and try a new .... or treatment. Some of these drugs have not yet been approved by international .... Sometimes the drugs are currently available ...., but are being tested for a new disease or additional information.
Most clinical trials that involve the .... of a new drug follow a series of steps, called .... This process allows researchers to ask and answer questions in a way that results in reliable information about the drug and protects the ....
Clinical trials are usually classified into one of four phases:

- In Phase I trials, researchers test a new drug or treatment in a .... group of people (20-80) for the first time to evaluate its safety, determine a safe dosage range, and identify ....
- In Phase II trials, the study drug or treatment is given to a .... group of people (100-300) to see if it is effective and to further evaluate its ....

- In Phase III trials, the study drug or treatment is given to large groups of people (1,000-3,000) to confirm its ...., monitor side effects, compare it to commonly used treatments, and collect information that will allow the drug or treatment to be used ....
- In Phase IV trials, post marketing studies delineate additional information including the drug's ...., benefits, and optimal use.

The success of clinical trials depends upon the participation of patients who volunteer. Participants in clinical trials can play a more active role in their own .... care, gain access to new research .... before they are widely available, and help others by contributing to medical ....

Exercise 9

Give a suitable English version to the following sentences.

1. Le persone partecipano come volontari ai test clinici per diverse ragioni.

   ....

   ....

2. Le persone non dovrebbero, comunque, entrare a far parte di un test clinico semplicemente perché una potenziale cura viene offerta gratuitamente.

   ....

   ....

3. I rischi dipendono dalla cura studiata in quel momento e dallo stato di salute delle persone che prendono parte al test.

   ....

   ....

Exercise 10

Give the Italian for:

1. Bias ....
2. Healthy ....
3. Device ....
4. Volunteering ....
5. Effective ....
6. Side effects ....

UNIT 2

THE WORLD OF PHARMACEUTICAL INDUSTRY

PHARMACEUTICAL COMPANIES

Most of today's major pharmaceutical companies were founded in the late 19th and early 20th centuries. Key discoveries of the 1920s and 1930s, such as insulin and penicillin, became mass-manufactured and distributed.

Legislation was enacted to test and approve drugs and to require appropriate labeling. Prescription and nonprescription drugs became legally distinguished from one another as the pharmaceutical industry matured. The industry got underway in earnest from the 1950s, due to the development of systematic scientific approaches, understanding of human biology (including DNA) and sophisticated manufacturing techniques.

Many new drugs were developed during the 1950s and mass-produced and marketed through the 1960s. This included the first oral contraceptive, "The Pill", cortisone, blood-pressure drugs and other heart medications. MAO inhibitors, chlorpromazine (Thorazine), haloperidol (Haldol) and the tranquilizers ushered in the age of psychiatric medication. Valium (diazepam), discovered in 1960, was marketed from 1963 and rapidly became the most prescribed drug in history, prior to controversy over dependency and habituation.

Attempts were made to increase regulation and to limit financial links between pharmaceutical companies and prescribing physicians, including by the relatively new US FDA. An increase in these attempts took place in the 1960s after the thalidomide tragedy came to light, in which the use of a new tranquilizer in pregnant women caused severe birth defects. In 1964, the World Medical Association issued its Declaration of Helsinki, which set standards for clinical research and demanded that subjects give their informed consent before enrolling in an experiment. Pharmaceutical companies became required to prove efficacy in clinical trials before marketing drugs.

Cancer drugs were a feature of the 1970s. From 1978, India took over as the primary center of pharmaceutical production without patent protection.

The industry remained relatively small scale until the 1970s when it began to expand at a greater rate. By the mid-1980s, small biotechnology firms were struggling for survival, which led to the formation of mutually beneficial partnerships with large pharmaceutical companies and a host of corporate buyouts of the

The Declaration of Helsinki was developed by the World Medical Association (WMA), as a set of ethical principles for the medical community relative to the experimentation in human, and although it is not a legally binding document it is regarded as the source of cornerstone principles to adopt in human research ethics.
The Declaration of Helsinki has been adopted by several times, the last one during the 59th WMA General Assembly, Seoul, October 2008. The text of the Declaration of Helsinki can be found at www.wma.net/en/30publications/10policies/b3/index.html

smaller firms. Pharmaceutical manufacturing became concentrated, with a few large companies holding a dominant position throughout the world and with a few companies producing medicines within each country.
The pharmaceutical industry entered the 1980s pressured by economics and a host of new regulations, both safety and environmental, but also transformed by new DNA chemistries and new technologies for analysis and computation. Drugs for heart disease and for AIDS were a feature of the 1980s, involving challenges to regulatory bodies and a faster approval process.
A new business atmosphere became institutionalized in the 1990s, characterized by mergers and takeovers, and by a dramatic increase in the use of contract research organizations for clinical development and even for basic R&D. The pharmaceutical industry confronted a new business climate and new regulations, born in part from dealing with world market forces and protests by activists in developing countries. Animal Rights activism was also a problem.

Big Pharma

Roughly half of the largest drug companies are based in Europe. (The exact count shifts because of mergers.) In 2002, the top ten were the American companies Pfizer, Merck, Johnson & Johnson, Bristol-Myers Squibb, and Wyeth (formerly American Home Products); the British companies GlaxoSmithKline and AstraZeneca; the Swiss companies Novartis and Roche; and the French company Aventis (which in 2004 merged with another French company, Sanofi Synthelabo, putting it in third place). Effective October 15, 2009 Pfizer acquired Wyeth in a cash and stock merger.
All are much alike in their operations.

Marketing changed dramatically in the 1990s, partly because of a new consumerism. The Internet made possible the direct purchase of medicines by drug consumers and of raw materials by drug producers, transforming the nature of business. In the US, Direct-to-consumer advertising proliferated on radio and TV because of new FDA regulations in 1997 that liberalized requirements for the presentation of risks. The new antidepressants, the SSRIs, notably fluoxetine (Prozac), rapidly became bestsellers and marketed for additional disorders.
Drug development progressed from a hit-and-miss approach to rational drug discovery in both laboratory design and natural-product surveys. Demand for nutritional supplements and so-called alternative medicines created opportunities and increased competition in the industry.

Functional Foods

Plant foods, such as fruits, vegetables, and whole grains contain many components that are beneficial to human health. Research supports that some of these foods, as part of an overall healthful diet, have the potential to delay the onset of many age-related diseases. These observations have led to continuing research aimed at identifying specific bioactive components in foods, so called "functional foods", which may be responsible for improving and maintaining health.
People should not automatically assume that consuming "functional foods" – also called "phoods" to suggest pharmaceuticals – will allow them to live longer, healthier lives. In a society that already has a ready stock of healthy fruits and vegetables, flocking to "functional foods" may bring no additional benefits. Some enhanced foods are useful for segments of the population with unique nutritional needs, such as vegans, who won't drink milk and need to find their calcium elsewhere. In other cases, such as prune juice laced with Lutein, the evidence supporting the benefits of the added nutrient is weak. For the general population, factors such as the overall nutritional value and calorie intake of your diet – as well, of course, as whether sound scientific evidence backs the claims on the package labels – should be considered before incorporating these foods into your routine. In addition, consumers should be aware that certain nutrients can interact with prescription or over-the-counter drugs. For example, calcium-fortified orange juice can decrease the effectiveness of some antibiotics.

Controversies emerged around adverse effects, notably regarding Vioxx in the US, and marketing tactics. Pharmaceutical companies became increasingly accused of disease mongering or over-medicalizing personal or social problems.
There are now more than 200 major pharmaceutical companies, jointly said to be more profitable than almost any other industry.

OFF-LABEL

Off-label use is the practice of prescribing drugs for a purpose outside the scope of the drug's approved purposes, most often concerning the drug's indication. In the United States, the Food and Drug Administration (FDA) requires numerous clinical trials to prove a drug's safety and efficacy in treating a given disease or condition. If satisfied that the drug is safe and effective, the drug's manufacturer and the FDA agree on specific language describing dosage, route and other information to be included on the drug's label. More detail is included in the drug's package insert. However, once the FDA approves a drug for prescription use, they do not attempt to regulate the practice of medicine, and so the physician makes decisions based on her or his best judgment. It is entirely legal in the United States and in many other countries to use drugs off-label. Exceptions to this are certain controlled substances, such as opiates, which cannot be legally prescribed except for approved purposes in the US. In Australia, amphetamines are included in these drugs, which cannot be prescribed off-label.
Some drugs are used more frequently off-label than for their original, FDA-approved indications.
Frequently the standard of care for a particular type or stage of cancer involves the off-label use of one or more drugs. An example is the use of tricyclic antidepressants to treat neuropathic pain. This old class of antidepressants is now rarely used for clinical depression due to side effects, but the tricyclics are often effective for treating pain.

A medical prescription is a written order by a qualified health care professional to a pharmacist or other therapist for a treatment to be provided to their patient. A prescription is a legal document which not only instructs in the preparation and provision of the medicine or device but indicates the prescriber takes responsibility for the clinical care of the patient and the outcomes that may or may not be achieved.

Pay attention

Labelling (British English) ➢ **Labeling** (American English)
Labelled " **Labeled** "

The 1960s ➢ the years from 1960 to 1969

Il **genitivo sassone** indica una relazione di possesso ed è dato da:
possessore + S + cosa posseduta
Dr. Reed's report.

Di norma il possessore dovrebbe essere una persona o un animale ma è diffuso l'uso del genitivo sassone anche in espressioni di tempo o quando il possessore non è una persona.
Body's key regulators the world's most prescribed drug.
Today's mail.

Exercise 1

Decide which statements are true (T) or false (F).

	T	F
1. A drug label contains all the possible details.		
2. The "off-label" use of drugs is considered illegal in US.		
3. A drug is used "off-label" when prescribed for purposes which are different from those suggested and approved.		
4. Opiates and amphetamines cannot be prescribed for "off-label" use in Australia.		
5. Cancer patients often receive drugs for an off-label indication.		
6. The use of tricyclics as pain relievers is "off-label".		

Exercise 2

Read the text on page 10 again and then fill in the blanks.

Legislation was enacted to test and approve drugs and to require .... labeling. Prescription and nonprescription drugs became legally .... from one another as the pharmaceutical industry matured. The industry got underway in earnest from the 1950s, due to the .... of systematic scientific approaches, understanding of human biology (including DNA) and sophisticated .... techniques.
The industry remained relatively .... until the 1970s when it began to expand at a greater .... By the mid-1980s, small biotechnology firms were struggling for survival, which led to the formation of mutually beneficial .... with large pharmaceutical companies and a host of corporate .... of the smaller firms.
Drugs for heart disease and for AIDS were a .... of the 1980s, involving challenges to regulatory bodies and a faster approval process.
Marketing changed dramatically in the 1990s, partly because of a new ....
The Internet made possible the direct .... of medicines by drug consumers and of .... by drug producers, transforming the nature of ....
Drug .... progressed from a hit-and-miss approach to rational drug discovery in both laboratory design and natural-product surveys. Demand for nutritional .... and so-called alternative medicines created new opportunities and .... competition in the industry.

WORD FILE

- **Buyout:** a situation where a person or group buys all the shares belonging to a company and so gets control of it.
- **Company:** a business organization that makes or sells goods or services. *Business:* firm. *To run a company:* to manage. *To set a company:* to start up. *To join a company:* to become an employee.
- **Consumerism:** the state of an advanced industrial society in which a lot of goods are for sale.

- **Disorder:** confusion, an illness of the mind or of the body.
- **Environment:** the air, water and land in or on which people, animals and plants live.
- **Mass-production:** to produce a lot of goods cheaply using machines in a factory.
- **Merger:** when two or more companies join together.
- **Patent:** the official legal right to exclusively make or sell an invention for a particular number of years.
- **Small scale:** describes an event or activity that is small in size.
- **Takeover:** when a company gets control of another company by buying most of its shares.
- **Vegan:** a person who doesn't eat meat, fish, eggs, cheese and doesn't use animal products such as leather.

- **Develop (to):** sviluppare.
- **Enroll (to):** ingaggiare,arruolare,registrare.
- **Feature:** caratteristica.
- **Hit-and-miss:** a casaccio.
- **Host:** gran numero di..., ospite.
- **Nutritional supplements:** integratori alimentari.
- **Raw materials:** materie prime.
- **Struggle for survival:** combattere per la sopravvivenza.
- **Usher(to):** far strada, introdurre.

Pay attention

Effective ➢ efficace, with a satisfactory outcome.
Effectively ➢ efficacemente (*He was a very effective speaker*).
In effect ➢ in practice.

Exercise 3

Match the definitions with the words in the box. (Pay attention! The given words are more than what you need.)

• label • merger • partnership • small-scale • mass production
• takeover • feature • patent • disorder • harm • goal

1. A piece of paper or another material that is attached to something and gives information about it.

   ....

2. When products are made in large numbers by machines so that they can be sold cheaply.

   ....

3. Involving only a small number of things or a small area.

   ....

4. The state of being a partner in business/a business owned by two or more people.

   ....

5. The joining together of two or more companies or organizations to form a larger one.

   ....

6. When one company takes control of another by buying more than half its shares.

   ....

Exercise 4

Fill in the table with short descriptions using the text on page 10.

1920s 1930s	
1950s	
1963	
1964	
1970s	
1978	
1990s	

ZERO TOLERANCE FOR COUNTERFEIT MEDICINES

Counterfeit medicines, already widespread in the developing world, are now found increasingly in the EU. While Internet-based sales are the main source of counterfeit medicines, these products are also appearing in the traditional supply chain. Urgent measures are required to protect European patients, including a ban on medicine repackaging.

Counterfeits have been found to contain toxic substances. Others contain no active ingredient, or the wrong amount of it – damaging to any medical treatment, but dangerous when patients are treated for serious illness. In most cases, it is impossible for the non-expert eye to distinguish the fakes from the originals.

Under current EU rules, products can be re-boxed, re-labelled or over-stickered. Tablets can be removed from their blisters and reconditioned. These repackaging activities can involve removing the security seal and damaging unique identification codes, which ensure product traceability. Such practices make it even harder to distinguish real medicines from fakes.

In addition to the development of security features on medicine packaging, individual companies assist authorities in different ways, for example by training officials to recognize fakes and by assisting with international police investigations. However, these initiatives alone are not enough.

The focus of the forthcoming EU legislative reform will be able to ensure that the integrity of the original package is absolutely guaranteed throughout the entire supply chain, from the time it leaves the original manufacturer to the point that it reaches the end user. This is a prerequisite for an effective anti-counterfeiting strategy.

In addition, liabilities will be more clearly defined for all involved in the distribution chain, including brokers, traders and agents. Heavy penalties will be enforced for trafficking in counterfeits. Efforts to set up a harmonized EU-wide identification system for medicines are encouraging.

[From www.efpia.org]

The "Pharmaceutical Package" is the popular name for a series of measures proposed by the European Commission impacting the pharmaceutical industry. This series included the "Communication on the future of the single market in pharmaceuticals for human use", which set out the Commissions's vision for the sector. The "Pharmaceutical Package" contains three important initiatives: a proposal for a directive on how to modernize pharmacovigilance in order to improve safety of medicines; a proposal to improve patient safety by reducing the infiltration of counterfeit medicines into the supply chain; and a directive on the future direction of the supply of health information to patients.

About EFPIA
EFPIA represents the pharmaceutical industry operating in Europe. Through its direct membership of 32 national associations and 43 leading pharmaceutical companies, EFPIA is the voice on the EU scene of 2,200 companies committed to researching, developing and bringing to patients new medicines that improve health .
For more information about EFPIA's position on Counterfeits www.efpia.org.

Exercise 5

Answer the following questions.

1. Which is the main source for the sale of counterfeit drugs?

   ....

   ....

2. Are counterfeits easy to be discovered?

   ....

   ....

3. Are current EU rules able to protect patients against fakes?

   ....

   ....

4. What can be considered a "prerequisite" for an anti-counterfeiting strategy?

   ....

   ....

5. Why a ban on medicine repackaging is so important?

   ....

   ....

Exercise 6

Give the Italian for.

1. The forthcoming EU legislative reform ....
2. A harmonized EU-wide identification system ....
3. Re-boxed, re-labelled or over-stickered ....
4. Medicine packaging ....
5. Internet based sales ....

Exercise 7

Read the text below and decide when the statements are true (T) or false (F).

The granting of the orphan drug status is designed to encourage the development of drugs which are necessary but would be prohibitively expensive/un-profitable to develop under normal circumstances.

In the United States, an orphan drug is any drug developed under the Orphan Drug Act of January 1983 (ODA), a federal law concerning rare diseases ("orphan diseases"), defined as diseases affecting fewer than 200,000 people in the United States or having a prevalence of less than 5 per 10,000 in the community. This has been adopted as a subclause of the Food and Drug Administration (FDA) regulations. Because medical research and development of drugs to treat such diseases is financially disadvantageous, companies that do so are rewarded with tax reductions and marketing exclusivity (a "monopoly") on that drug for an extended time (seven years post-approval). The concept behind the ODA is that the longer period of exclusivity will encourage more companies to invest money in research. Under the act many drugs have been developed, including drugs to treat glioma, multiple myeloma, cystic fibrosis, and snake venom. In the US, from January 1983 to June 2004, a total of 1,129 different orphan drug designations have been granted by the Office of Orphan Products Development (OOPD) and 249 orphan drugs have received marketing authorization in the US. In contrast, the decade prior to 1983 saw fewer than ten such products come to market.

A similar status exists in the European Union, administered by the Committee on Orphan Medicinal Products of the European Medicines Agency.

In 2003, the leading orphan drug by worldwide sales revenue was Amgen's Erythropoietin (Epogen®), with sales of $2.4bn.

		T	F
1.	The ODA is a federal law.	▢	▢
2.	When a disease affects more than 200,000 people it is called orphan disease.	▢	▢
3.	A tax reward is granted to companies which carry out research and development of drugs treating orphan diseases.	▢	▢
4.	The ODA wants to increase investments in research thanks to tax reductions for companies.	▢	▢
5.	The benefit of this federal law lasted from January 1983 to June 2004.	▢	▢
6.	In this period 1,129 medicines have been designed as orphan drugs.	▢	▢
7.	No European law can be considered similar to the American ODA.	▢	▢
8.	Amgen's Erythropoietin was at the top of the 2003 orphan drug sales.	▢	▢

UNIT 3

DRUGS

LIPITOR

Before taking any medicine, it's good to know how it works. LIPITOR is a statin. Statins lower cholesterol in your body. They block an enzyme in the liver. Your body uses this enzyme to make cholesterol. When less cholesterol is made, the liver uses more of it from the blood. This results in lower levels of cholesterol in your blood.
LIPITOR is clinically proven to lower bad cholesterol 39-60%, when diet and exercise aren't enough (average effect depending on dose).
As the #1 prescribed cholesterol-lowering medication in the world, over 26 million people in the United States have been prescribed LIPITOR.
LIPITOR has been studied in more than 400 completed and ongoing studies. These studies include over 80,000 patients.

- In clinical studies of 2500 LIPITOR patients, 98% did not have side effects that caused them to stop taking their medicine.
- A landmark study found that LIPITOR reduced the risk of heart attack, stroke, certain kinds of heart surgeries, and chest pain in patients with several common risk factors for heart disease.
- Another landmark study found that LIPITOR significantly reduces the risk of heart attack and stroke in patients with both type 2 diabetes and at least 1 other risk factor for heart disease.

Three times more cardiologists surveyed would recommend LIPITOR to their own family members over other cholesterol lowering drugs.

Pfizer Worldwide

Pfizer Inc. is a research-based, global pharmaceutical company that was founded in the US by two German immigrants, Charles Pfizer and Charles Erhart, in 1849. Today, Pfizer is continuously discovering, developing, manufacturing and marketing leading prescription-only medicines for humans and animals as well as a wide portfolio of consumer healthcare products. Currently, Pfizer employs over 120,000 people in more than 60 countries and has sales in over 150 countries. Pfizer has major US R&D sites in New London & Groton (Connecticut), La Jolla (California), Ann Arbor (Michigan), with major international sites in Toronto (Canada), Sandwich (United Kingdom), Nagoya (Japan) and Fresnes (France). It also has at least 28 additional clinical research sites worldwide. In 2004, overall investment in R&D is estimated at about $8 billion – the largest investment of any pharmaceutical company and of any private sector research institution in the world.

Pay attention

At least ➢ almeno, come minimo
Little ➢ less (comparativo di magg.) ➢ the least (superlativo)

Exercise 1

Fill in the following table about LIPITOR.

How it works	
Number of trials	
Side effects-free percentage	
Benefits	

Exercise 2

Fill in the blanks with the words from the box.

• to stop • medicine • has been studied • uses • disease • ongoing • liver
• have been prescribed • to lower •is made • at least • pain • side effects • reduced • enough

Before taking any ...., it's good to know how it works. LIPITOR is a statin. Statins lower cholesterol in your body.

They block an enzyme in the .... Your body .... this enzyme to make cholesterol. When less cholesterol ...., the liver uses more of it from the blood. This results in lower levels of cholesterol in your blood.

LIPITOR is clinically proved .... bad cholesterol 39-60%, when diet and exercise aren't .... (average effect depending on dose).

As the first prescribed cholesterol-lowering medication in the world, over 26 million people in the United States .... LIPITOR.

LIPITOR .... in more than 400 completed and .... studies. These studies include over 80,000 patients.

- In clinical studies of 2500 LIPITOR patients, 98% did not have .... that caused them .... taking their medicine;
- a landmark study found that LIPITOR .... the risk of heart attack, stroke, certain kinds of heart surgeries, and chest .... in patients with several common risk factors for heart ....;
- another landmark study found that LIPITOR significantly reduces the risk of heart attack and stroke in patients with both type 2 diabetes and .... 1 other risk factor for heart disease.

BEING ON ZOMETA THERAPY

Zometa is an FDA-approved prescription drug developed by Novartis Oncology. It is used to treat patients with multiple myeloma. Zometa is also used to treat other cancers – including breast, lung and prostate cancer – that have spread to the bones, a process called bone metastasis. When cancer has spread to the bone, treatment with Zometa helps to protect bones and may reduce or delay such complications as:

- bone fracture;
- need for radiation and/or surgery to bone;
- spinal cord compression.

Even patients who have already experienced bone complications from the spread of cancer to the bones may be helped by treatment with Zometa.

Zometa is used with cancer treatments such as radiation, hormonal therapy, or chemotherapy.

If therapy with Zometa is recommended for you, here are some things you should know.

- Zometa is given as an intravenous infusion every 3 to 4 weeks. You may receive it at your doctor's office or at a clinic or infusion center. The infusion takes at least 15 minutes once Zometa is prepared.
- Concerns that you may have about receiving intravenous Zometa should be weighed against the potential benefits of treatment, as the complications of bone metastases can be devastating.
- While you are receiving treatment with Zometa, it is important to take certain dietary supplements daily. You should take a multivitamin that contains 400 IU of Vitamin D. You should also take an oral calcium supplement of at least 500 mg.
- In some cases, Zometa and other bisphosphonates have been known to cause kidney damage. Prior to each infusion, your doctor will routinely do blood tests or monitor your kidney function. If you have kidney problems, your doctor may determine that Zometa should be administered at a reduced dose or should not be given. Patients with severe kidney problems should not take Zometa.
- It is also important to keep up your fluid intake while on Zometa therapy. Signs and symptoms of low fluid intake include thirst, low urine output, and dry mouth. Be sure to drink plenty of water or other fluids.

Your doctor will closely watch your response to Zometa.

While taking Zometa, you may experience fatigue, nausea, vomiting, bone pain, headache, shortness of breath, or lack of appetite. When these adverse events were seen in patients taking Zometa, they were usually mild and transient. Your doctor can recommend a mild pain reliever to make you more comfortable.

Zometa should be used with caution in patients with aspirin-sensitive asthma. Zometa should not be given to women who are pregnant, because there is the potential that it might harm the fetus. Women given Zometa should not become pregnant during therapy.

Oral hygiene is very important for patients living with cancer. Some patients have reported problems with their jaw bones while being treated with Zometa please talk to your doctor before undergoing invasive dental procedures such as tooth extractions or if you experience pain in your jaw or poor wound healing in your mouth.

Pay attention

Tooth extraction	Prescription drugs
Pain reliever	Heart medications
Blood pressure levels	Treatment goals
High blood pressure medications	Drugs safety information

Sono parole composte dove dei sostantivi assumono la valenza di aggettivi. Questi ultimi diventano invariabili.

Exercise 3

Decide which statements are true (T) or false (F).

	T	F
1. Zometa is suggested in case of lung cancer.		
2. In some cases Zometa can reduce the need for radiation.		
3. Patients are recommended to take Zometa every 3 or 4 weeks.		
4. Patients are suggested not to take any vitamin or calcium supplement.		
5. Researchers have realized that Zometa can cause kidney damages.		
6. Signs and symptoms of low fluid intake highlight severe kidney problems.		
7. Patients with shortness of breath shouldn't be given Zometa.		
8. Oral calcium supplements are recommended in case of adverse events such as fatigue and bone pain.		
9. Patients may experience pain in their jaw bones.		

Exercise 4

Answer the following questions following the given suggestions.

1. How is Zometa given to patients?
   Patients are supposed ....
2. Can patients be treated with Zometa at their home?
   No, they can't. They are ....
3. Do patients treated with Zometa have to take care about their diet?
   Yes, they do. They are suggested ....
4. Which symptoms must suggest patients to drink a lot?
   The signs shown by patients include ....
5. Why blood tests should be done before each infusion?
   Because blood tests can show ....
6. In which cases Zometa is not suggested?
   When patients have ....
   This drug may have effects such as ....
7. What can a doctor prescribe patients in case of adverse effects?
   Doctors can prescribe ....
8. What is a "bone metastasis"?
   It is a process by which the cancer ....

Exercise 5

Read this text and decide which statements are true (T) or false (F).

Basel, January 20, 2010 – Patients in Japan will benefit from the approval of three new Novartis medicines – Equa marketed as Galvus in the European Union, for the treatment of type 2 diabetes,

Exforge for high blood pressure, and Afinitor for advanced kidney cancer. These approvals reinforce the strong commitment of Novartis to helping patients in Japan, the company's second-largest pharmaceutical market.

Equa has been approved in Japan for the treatment of type 2 diabetes, as monotherapy or in combination with a sulfonylurea. As a DPP-4 inhibitor, Equa works by targeting the dysfunction in the pancreatic islets that causes high blood sugar levels in people with type 2 diabetes.

Equa has been approved for doses of 50 mg twice daily, or 50 mg once daily, depending on the needs of the individual patient. Patients treated with Equa 50 mg twice daily demonstrated an average reduction in HbA1c – a marker of blood glucose level – of 1.2% compared to placebo, which would bring half of them within the maximum HbA1c value of 6.5% recommended by the Japan Diabetes Society. Equa was shown to be well-tolerated with a favorable profile in terms of hypoglycemia and bodyweight.

An estimated 7 million people in Japan have type 2 diabetes and approximately 70% of patients are still not meeting their HbA1c goals on their current medications. When left untreated or inadequately controlled, type 2 diabetes can lead to heart and kidney disease, blindness, and vascular or neurologic problems.

[Novartis Oncology, adapted from]

		T	F
1.	Equa is available only on the Japanese market.	■	■
2.	Equa's aim is treating pancreatic islets dysfunctions.	■	■
3.	Clinical trials proved Equa provide a HbA1c value of 6.5% in patients treated with a 50 mg daily.	■	■
4.	The Equa daily dose depends on the needs of each patient.	■	■
5.	A large part of Japanese people with type 2 diabetes reach values under 6.5%.	■	■
6.	Blindness can occur in patients with type 2 diabetes not properly treated.	■	■

WORD FILE

- **Blood:** the red liquid that your heart pumps around your body. *To bleed, bled, bled:* to lose blood (*Your nose is bleeding*).
- **Chest:** the front part of your body between your neck and your stomach.
- **Enzyme:** a catalytic substance, protein in nature, formed by living cells and having a specific action in promoting a chemical change.
- **Harm (to):** to physically hurt a person or animal (to damage something).
- **Inhibitor:** a substance that checks or stops a chemical action.
- **Jaw:** one of the two bones that your teeth are in. Upper/lower jaw.
- **Kidney:** one of the two organs in your lower back that filter waste products from your blood and produce urine.
- **Lung:** one of the two organs in your body that allow breathing.
- **Statin:** a drug that is used to lower cholesterol and reduce the risk of getting heart disease.
- **Wound:** an injury to your body often caused by a knife or a bullet (*It'll take some days for your wounds to heal. The nurse bandaged the wound*).

- **Achieve (to):** raggiungere, realizzare, ottenere.
- **Aim:** mira, obiettivo, intenzione, congettura.
- **Compare with or to (to):** paragonare.
- **Exciting:** emozionante.
- **Forefront:** prima linea, avanguardia.
- **Goal:** traguardo, meta, scopo.
- **Heal (to):** sanare.
- **Heart attack:** attacco cardiaco.
- **Heart failure:** insufficienza cardiaca.
- **Heart stroke:** colpo, pulsazione cardiaca.
- **Landmark:** caratteristica, punto di riferimento, pietra miliare.

TEKTURNA, FIRST NEW TYPE OF ANTIHYPERTENSIVE DRUG

New study results show more patients receiving both Tekturna and Diovan reached target blood pressure goal compared to those taking either agent alone.
Tekturna, approved in the US as first direct renin inhibitor, works by directly targeting an enzyme which triggers a process that can lead to high blood pressure.
Tekturna provides significant blood pressure reductions for a full 24 hours and is generally well tolerated.
There is urgent need for new therapies like Tekturna since nearly 70% of patients with high blood pressure are still not achieving treatment goals.
Basel, March 26, 20.. – Results from a new study have shown patients taking two Novartis cardiovascular medicines – the recently US-approved drug Tekturna® (aliskiren) and the leading therapy Diovan® (valsartan) – experienced greater reductions in blood pressure levels than those using either agent alone.
The study also found more patients receiving both Tekturna, which received US approval in March and represents the first type of new high blood pressure medicine in a decade, and Diovan reached their treatment goal compared to either drug alone.
Data from this trial involving 1,800 patients – the first large-scale study to assess the benefits of combining these medicines – were presented for the first time at the American College of Cardiology 56th Scientific Session in New Orleans.
Half of the patients in the eight-week trial taking both Tekturna and Diovan saw a reduction in blood pressure to the target of 140/90 mmHg (systolic/diastolic pressure), higher levels than seen in patients taking either of the medicines alone. Failure to properly control high blood pressure, also called hypertension, can increase the risk of heart attacks and strokes.
Tekturna and Diovan work in different ways to target the Renin Angiotensin System, one of the body's key regulators of blood pressure. Tekturna targets renin, an enzyme responsible for triggering a process that can lead to high blood pressure. Diovan, an angiotensin receptor blocker (ARB) and one of the world's most-prescribed cardiovascular medicines, blocks a hormone later in this system that causes narrowing of blood vessels.
"These study results are exciting because they suggest the value of different mechanisms of action when Tekturna and Diovan are used together", said Suzanne Oparil, MD, Director of the Vascular Biology and Hypertension Program and Professor of Medicine at the University of Alabama at Birmingham in Alabama.

"In addition to important blood pressure lowering, the combination of Tekturna and Diovan maintained a tolerability profile similar to that seen with either agent alone" , Dr. Oparil said.

Tekturna received US regulatory approval for treatment of high blood pressure as monotherapy or in combination with other high blood pressure medications. In an extensive clinical trial program involving more than 6,400 patients, Tekturna provided significant blood pressure reductions for a full 24 hours. This once-daily oral therapy is expected to be available by the end of March in US pharmacies as 150 mg and 300 mg tablets.

A second study presented at the meeting compared Tekturna to Ramipril, another high blood pressure medicine in a class known as ACE inhibitors. Results showed more patients treated with the Tekturna-based therapy reached their blood pressure goal than patients treated with the ramipril-based therapy (61.4% vs. 53.1% respectively).

The need for new high blood pressure medicines is urgent given that this condition affects one in four adults globally and more than 70% of these patients remain uncontrolled. In fact, many require two or more medications to reach their target blood pressure goal. Uncontrolled high blood pressure can increase the risk of cardiovascular disease, the world's leading cause of death.

Exercise 6

Decide which statements are true (T) or false (F).

		T	F
1.	Tekturna used with Diovan provides a further reduction of blood pressure.	■	■
2.	New studies compared patients taking Tekturna with others taking Diovan.	■	■
3.	Tekturna works by targeting an enzyme which is responsible for high blood pressure.	■	■
4.	The 70% of patient with high blood pressure get easily significant blood pressure reduction.	■	■
5.	Tekturna can provide greater reductions in blood pressure than Diovan.	■	■
6.	The 1,800 patient involved in the Novartis study had the goal of 140/90 mmHg.	■	■
7.	Hypertension means low blood pressure.	■	■
8.	The daily oral therapy of Tekturna provides a 24 hours blood pressure reduction.	■	■
9.	Tekturna is an ACE inhibitor.	■	■

Exercise 7

Fill in the gaps with a suitable word from the passage.

1. It .... a significant blood pressure reduction.
2. The first .... scale study to .... the benefits of combining these medicines.
3. Half of the .... in the eight week .... taking both Tekturna and Diovan saw a reduction in .... pressure.

4. In .... to important blood pressure lowering, the two medicines maintained a .... profile similar to that seen with .... agent alone.
5. High blood pressure can .... the risk of cardiovascular diseases.
6. This once .... oral therapy is expected .... by the end of March in US ....

Exercise 8

Find the requested words in the passage.

1. The opposite of low. ....
2. The opposite of last. ....
3. A synonym of aim. ....
4. The opposite of unexciting. ....
5. A synonym of advantage. ....
6. A synonym of earlier. ....
7. A synonym of ill person. ....
8. The opposite of decrease. ....
9. A synonym of supply. ....
10. The opposite of different. ....
11. A synonym of main cause. ....
12. A synonym of tension. ....

Exercise 9

Read this text and answer the questions.

Aspirin

Aspirin®, or acetylsalicylic acid is a salicylate drug often used as an analgesic, antipyretic, and as an anti-inflammatory. It also has an antiplatelet effect and is used in long-term, low doses to prevent heart attacks and blood clot formation in people at high risk for developing blood clots.
High doses of aspirin may also be given immediately after an acute heart attack; these doses may inhibit the synthesis of prothrombin and therefore produce a second and different anticoagulant effect, although this is not well understood.
The main undesirable side effects of aspirin are gastrointestinal distress – including ulcers and stomach bleeding – and tinnitus, especially in higher doses. Another adverse effect is increased bleeding in menstruating women, due to aspirin's anticoagulant properties. In children under 12 years of age, aspirin is no longer used to control flu-like symptoms or the symptoms of chickenpox, due to the risk of Reye's syndrome.
Aspirin was the first-discovered member of the class of drugs known as non-steroidal anti inflammatory drugs (NSAIDs), not all of which are salicylates, although they all have similar effects and most have some mechanism of action which involves non-selective inhibition of the enzyme cyclooxygenase.

1. In which cases Aspirin can be suggested to patients?

....

....

....

2. Which are the main side effects?

....

....

....

3. Which class of drugs is Aspirin the first discovered member?

....

....

....

Exercise 10

Read this Media Release from the University of Bath and decide which statements are true (T) or false (F).

Professor Corinne de Vries from the University of Bath's Department of Pharmacy & Pharmacology has urged diabetes patients not to stop taking their medication without consulting their doctor following research suggesting a link between the drug rosiglitazone and an increased risk of heart failure.

Research published in the British Medical Journal (BMJ) suggests that rosiglitazone (Avandia), a drug used to treat type 2 diabetes, is associated with an increased risk of heart failure and death among older patients compared to a similar drug, pioglitazone.

However, Professor de Vries, Professor of Pharmacoepidemiology, has written in an accompanying editorial that the data in the study do not fully support the claim that pioglitazone should be favoured over rosiglitazone.

De Vries said that patients taking rosiglitazone were sicker than those taking pioglitazone, so these patients were more likely to develop heart failure.

She said: "The data presented by the Canadian study do not support the suggestion that you should favor one drug over the other.There is no reason to believe yet that there is a difference."

Rosiglitazone and pioglitazone belong to a class of drugs called thiazolidinediones and are widely used for the treatment of type 2 diabetes. They help to control blood sugar levels, but both drugs can also cause side effects including weight gain, fluid retention and heart failure.

In the study published in the BMJ, researchers in Canada compared the risk of heart attack, heart failure and death in patients treated with rosiglitazone and pioglitazone.

Using prescription records, they identified nearly 40,000 patients aged 66 years and older who started treatment with either rosiglitazone or pioglitazone between April 2002 and March 2008.

Data on hospital admission for either a heart attack or heart failure during the six-year study period were recorded and deaths were identified from a national database.

Detailed analysis showed that patients treated with pioglitazone had a significantly lower risk of heart failure and death compared to patients treated with rosiglitazone, but there was no significant difference in the risk of heart attack.

The study estimated that, for every 93 patients treated with rosiglitazone rather than pioglitazone, one additional cardiovascular event or death would be predicted to occur annually.

But whilst the study reinforces the message that thiazolidinediones should be avoided in heart failure patients, Professor De Vries cautioned that further research was needed to determine a full risk-benefit profile for the medicine.
She said: "Nobody should stop taking their medication without consulting their doctor."
People who have concerns regarding their diabetes treatment are urged to consult their GP and not to discontinue taking their medication.

	T	F
1. Diabetes patients are suggested to be more likely to have heart failure owing to the use of a drug.	■	■
2. The discussion is based on the study of the side effects of the two drugs.	■	■
3. Patients taking drugs for diabetes often get weight.	■	■
4. The study was carried out by the University of Bath researchers who used hospital data and prescription records.	■	■
5. Professor de Vries completely agrees and supports the research published on the British Medical Journal.	■	■
6. The study showed that patients taking Rosiglitazone had an increased risk of heart failure and death.	■	■
7. Patients with heart diseases or disorders should avoid thiazolidinediones medicines.	■	■
8. Diabetes patients are urged to consult their GP and to stop taking their medicines.	■	■
9. This research was published on a newspaper.	■	■

WORD FILE

- **Blood vessels:** the tubes through which the blood flows in your body.
- **Chickenpox:** an acute contagious disease caused by herpes varicella zoster virus.
- **Hypertension:** excessive tension or pressure in bodily fluids such as blood.
- **Renin:** a proteolytic enzyme in kidney that acts on renin substrate to liberate angiotensin.
- **Tinnitus:** a ringing or booming sensation in one or both ears; a symptom of an ear infection.

- **Achieve (to):** raggiungere, realizzare. *Achievement*: raggiungimento.
- **Antiplatelet:** antipiastrinico.
- **Blood clot formation:** formazione di coaguli di sangue.
- **Fluid retention:** ritenzione idrica.
- **Leading:** principale, di grande importanza.
- **Lower (to):** abbassare.
- **Narrow (to):** restringere.
- **Product:** prodotto. *Produce:* rendimento, prodotto agricolo.
- **Target:** obiettivo, intenzione.
- **Target (to):** mirare a.
- **Trigger:** grilletto.
- **Trigger (to):** scatenare.
- **Urge (to):** esortare, raccomandare, insistere.
- **Weight gain:** aumento di peso.

UNIT 4

PHARMACOVIGILANCE

AN FDA STORY

In 1999, the United States Food and Drug Administration (FDA) approved Vioxx (known generically as rofecoxib), a Merck product for treating arthritis. Vioxx was stronger than existing medications, while easier on the stomach than established anti-inflammatory drugs such as naproxen. Vioxx became one of the most prescribed drugs in history. According to internal e-mail traffic released at a later lawsuit, Merck had a list of doctors critical of Vioxx to be "neutralised" or "discredited".

Thereafter, studies by Merck and by others found an increased risk of heart attack associated with Vioxx use when compared with naproxen. There was no indication of this risk in the original placebo-controlled safety trials, and it was possible that the effect was more related to naproxen decreasing the risk of heart attacks than one of Vioxx increasing the risk. Merck adjusted the labeling of Vioxx to reflect possible cardiovascular risks in 2002.

On September 23, 2004, Merck received information about results from a clinical trial it was conducting that included findings of increased risk of heart attacks among Vioxx users who had been using the medication for over eighteen months. On September 28, 2004, Merck notified the FDA that it was voluntarily withdrawing Vioxx from the market, and it publicly announced the withdrawal on September 30. The FDA has since recommended that Vioxx be put back on the market, but with a more prominent warning regarding cardiovascular risks on its label.

On November 5, 2004 the medical journal The Lancet published the results of its analysis of the available studies. It concluded that "the unacceptable cardiovascular risks of Vioxx (rofecoxib) were evident as early as 2000..." The journal's editors criticized Merck for having kept the drug on the market as long as it did before withdrawing it, and also criticized the FDA for its failure of regulatory oversight.

About 50,000 people have sued Merck claiming that they or their family members have suffered medical problems such as heart attacks or strokes after taking Vioxx. In 2005, Merck was found liable in the first case that went to trial and the plaintiff was awarded $253.4 million in damages; however, the judgement was subsequently reduced to $20 million and then, upon appeal, the verdict was reversed in 2008. In November 2007, Merck proposed to pay $4.85 billion to settle most of the pending Vioxx lawsuits. The settlement will require that claimants provide medical proof of having suffered a heart attack or a stroke and show they received at least 30 Vioxx pills. This proposed settlement is generally viewed by industry analysts and investors as a victory for Merck, considering that original estimates of Merck's liability reached as high as $50 billion. As of mid-2008, plaintiffs have

> **The Food and Drug Administration (FDA or USFDA) is an agency of the United States Department of Health and Human Services and is responsible for regulating and supervising the safety of foods, dietary supplements, drugs, vaccines, biological medical products, blood products, medical devices, radiation-emitting devices, veterinary products, and cosmetics.**

prevailed in only three of the twenty cases that have reached juries, all with relatively small awards. On May 20, 2008, Merck was found liable for using deceptive marketing tactics to promote Vioxx and 30 states will split the $58 million settlement. The amount is the largest multi-state settlement against a pharmaceutical company. All its new television pain-advertisements must be vetted by the Food and Drug Administration and changed or delayed upon request until 2018.

The Lancet is one of the world's best-known and most respected general medical journals, with editorial offices in London and New York, The Lancet was founded in 1823 by Thomas Wakley, who named it after the surgical instrument called a lancet, as well as an arched window ("to let in light").
The Lancet **has taken a stand on several important medical issues. Recent examples include criticism of the World Health Organization, rejecting claims of the efficacy of homeopathy as a therapeutic option, disapproval during the time Reed Exhibitions hosted arms industry fairs, and a call in 2003 for tobacco to be made illegal.**

Exercise 1

Decide which statements are true (T) or false (F).

		T	F
1.	Vioxx had a less strong effect on the stomach than Naproxen.	☐	☐
2.	Vioxx is known to have been a bestseller in prescription drugs.	☐	☐
3.	The safety trials proved a possible increasing risk of heart attacks by Vioxx.	☐	☐
4.	2002 Vioxx label warned about heart risks.	☐	☐
5.	Vioxx was obliged by the FDA to withdraw Vioxx from the market.	☐	☐
6.	The evidence of increased risk of strokes and heart attacks were notified to Merck in September 2004.	☐	☐
7.	The Lancet was critical towards the Merck Company and the FDA.	☐	☐
8.	Merck was found liable for causing heart attacks and asked to pay $253.4 million.	☐	☐
9.	Twenty cases proved the Merck's liability and all received small awards.	☐	☐
10.	Vioxx was obliged to pay $58 million as settlement for deceptive marketing.	☐	☐

WORD FILE

- **Claim (to):** pretendere, asserire, rivendicare.
- **Claimant:** richiedente
- **Damage:** danno.
- **Lawsuit:** azione legale, vertenza.
- **Liability:** responsabilità.
- **Oversight:** supervisione.
- **Plaintiff:** ricorrente, querelante.
- **Proof, evidence:** prova.
- **Settle (to):** accordarsi, saldare, sistemare, sistemarsi.
- **Settlement:** liquidazione, transazione, definizione.
- **Vet (to):** passare al vaglio.

BAYCOL

The Bayer pharmaceutical company in august 2001 withdrew its popular new statin drug Baycol (cerivastatin) from the market. Company executives felt constrained to take this radical move because an analysis of new data showed that 31 patients taking Baycol had died from a severe muscle disorder called rhabdomyolysis.

Rhabdomyolysis occurs when a large number of skeletal muscle cells die, thus releasing a massive amount of muscle protein into the bloodstream. This muscle protein becomes entrapped in the kidneys, essentially clogging up the filtering process of the kidneys and leading to kidney failure and other organ system disorders.

Rhabdomyolysis is extremely rare as a drug side effect. It is most commonly seen after massive muscle trauma (after an auto accident, for instance), or as a chief component of heat stroke – the condition that killed Minnesota Vikings star Korey Stringer. While all statin drugs are known to cause a low-grade muscle disorder in some patients – a disorder similar to rhabdomyolysis but on a much smaller scale – the report with Baycol was the first time a statin had been implicated in actually causing death by producing a severe muscle disorder.

As noted, all statins can and do cause problems with the skeletal muscles in some patients, and muscular pain is one of the more common reasons that statins must be discontinued in some individuals. However, it was recognized that Baycol had a much greater propensity for causing muscle problems than do the other statins, in fact, it is not at all clear that other statins can cause actual rhabdomyolysis. So while precautions need to be taken when using any statin the potentially fatal problem of rhabdomyolysis seems to be limited to Baycol.

Of the 31 people who died from Baycol-induced rhabdomyolysis, 12 were also taking gemfibrozil, another lipid-lowering agent. It has been known for some time that using statins in combination with gemfibrozil can make muscle problems more likely to occur, and the warning labeling for statin drugs have reflected this fact.

In the remaining 19 patients who died taking Baycol, it has been reported that the large majority were started directly on the highest dose of the drug. (The usual starting dose – and the recommended starting dose – was 0.4 mg. Most of the cases of rhabdomyolysis occurred after a 0.8 mg tablet was introduced in August 2000, when, apparently, many doctors took to prescribing the higher dose immediately).

In other words, if the prescribing practices of doctors had followed a more conservative (i.e., the recommended) path, it seems likely that most of these fatal cases of rhabdomyolysis might not have occurred. Indeed, Bayer withdrew Baycol from every country in the world except Japan – where gemfibrozil is not used, and where the 0.8 mg tablet is not available. The available data supports this decision.

For patients taking the more established statin drugs (lovastatin, simvastatin, pravastatin, and atorvastatin) the problems with Baycol should not create any additional concern. These older drugs have been used in hundreds of thousands of patients for more than a decade without causing similar problems. Thus, for these drugs the recommendations have not changed. Statins should generally not be used in combination with gemfibrozil – for reasons that are not at all clear, this com-

Pay attention

Data ➢ dati ➢ plurale non numerabile

i.e. ➢ from the latin "id est"
it means it is

bination of drugs greatly increases the risk of muscular disorders. Additionally, people taking statins who experience muscle aches and pains should report this symptom to their doctors. A simple blood test (the CPK level) should reveal whether the statin drug is causing any degree of skeletal muscle destruction – if so, the statin should be discontinued.

Exercise 2

Decide which statements are true (T) or false (F).

		T	F
1.	Patients died of a muscle disorder caused by a statin drug.	▢	▢
2.	Rhabdomyolysis causes a massive increase in the number of muscle cells.	▢	▢
3.	This disease happens in very rare cases.	▢	▢
4.	Statin drugs are known to be connected with some kind of minor muscle disorders.	▢	▢
5.	Baycol turned out not to be implicated in the death of patients caused by severe muscle disorder.	▢	▢
6.	All statin drugs need caution because often cause muscle diseases.	▢	▢
7.	It was unknown that statin drugs in combination with lipid-lowering agents could cause unwanted side effects.	▢	▢
8.	The Bayer Company was obliged to withdraw Baycol from every country in the world.	▢	▢

Exercise 3

Translate the words in italics.

For patients taking the more established statin drugs (lovastatin, simvastatin, pravastatin, and atorvastatin) the problems with Baycol *non dovrebbero creare ulteriori preoccupazioni*. These older drugs have been used in hundreds of thousands of patients *per più di un decennio* without causing similar problems. Thus, for these drugs the recommendations have not changed. Statins should generally not be used *unitamente a* gemfibrozil – for reasons that are not at all clear, this combination of drugs *aumenta notevolmente* the risk of muscular disorders. Additionally, people taking statins who experience muscle aches and pains dovrebbero *riferire questo sintomo* to their doctors. *Un semplice esame del sangue* (the CPK level) should reveal whether the statin drug is causing any degree of skeletal muscle destruction – if so, the statin *dovrebbe essere interrotta*.

....

....

....

WORD FILE

- **Kidney:** one of the two organs in your lower back that separate waste products from your body and make urine.
- **Skeleton:** the structure consisting in all the bones in a human or animal body. *Skeletal:* relating to the skeleton.
- **Statin:** a drug used to lower cholesterol reducing the risks of heart diseases.

Exercise 4

Answer the following questions.

1. Why was Baycol withdrawn from the market?

   ...

2. Which kind of disorder is rhabdomyolysis?

   ...

3. Is it a common drug side effect?

   ...

4. When is it more likely to occur?

   ...

5. Statin drugs can be considered "safe drugs"?

   ...

6. Why wasn't Baycol withdrawn from Japan?

   ...

7. How to investigate whether a statin drug is causing muscle disorders?

   ...

8. Did old statin drugs prove to be safe?

   ...

Adverse Drug Reactions Key Facts

- Unintended, harmful reactions to medicines (known as adverse drug reactions) are among the leading causes of death in many countries.
- The majority of adverse drug reactions (ADR) are preventable.
- People in every country of the world are affected by ADRs.
- In some countries ADR-related costs, such as hospitalization, surgery and lost productivity, exceed the cost of the medications.

No medicine is risk free. Vigilant assessment of the risks and benefits of medicines promotes patient safety.

HOW TO PREVENT ANOTHER VIOOX CASE

What could be done to prevent another Vioxx? This pain medication for arthritis became a blockbuster after its introduction in 1999, only to be taken off the market in 2004 when a study linked the drug to an increased risk of heart attack and strokes.

A study published in Archives of Internal Medicine offers an ambitious proposal to determine a drug's risks sooner than they might otherwise become evident. The authors propose a system to examine widely prescribed drugs through safety analyses that would pool data as they emerge from various clinical trials of a medication and aggregate the information for a fuller picture of a drug's harms and benefits.

As policy makers in Washington push for various forms of evidence gathering to determine the safety and effectiveness of medical treatments, the study proposes a broad model for monitoring drug safety that would consist of detailed publicly available data that independent researchers could freely analyze.

Such a database could be continually updated and aggregated with new information, as the results of new studies were published, to calculate a near real-time balance sheet of a drug's risks and benefits.

Dr. Joseph S. Ross, the lead author of the study, said the objective of the researchers was to determine whether this kind of sequential cumulative analysis could serve as a new model for monitoring the safety of drugs after they enter the market.

"How could we be doing post-market surveillance in a better way?" said Dr. Ross, an assistant professor of geriatrics and palliative medicine at Mount Sinai School of Medicine in Manhattan. "For drugs that we are concerned about, that are high risk, this could be a blueprint going forward."

Drug makers and researchers regularly conduct studies called meta-analyses in which they aggregate results from some previous studies of a drug, using the combined information to summarize the benefits and risks of a treatment. But the new study proposes a continuously updated model. Using data from Vioxx as their example, the researchers reported that Merck, the drug's maker, could have known about the increased cardiovascular risk several years earlier if the company had used the methodology.

The cumulative analysis of the researchers showed that by May 2002 – more than two years before Merck pulled Vioxx off the market – study patients on the drug had a 39 percent increased risk of heart attack or death compared with people taking a placebo.

Dr. Ross and his co-authors have each worked as paid consultants to plaintiffs involved in lawsuits against Merck over Vioxx injury claims. The researchers used documents obtained through the litigation, including detailed data from Merck's Vioxx studies, to conduct their analysis.

In a statement Monday, Merck questioned the methodology of the authors, saying that the researchers had used categories that were too broad. The researchers, for example, counted heart attacks and deaths that happened after patients had stopped taking Vioxx.

In 2000, a study financed by Merck had reported an increased cardiovascular risk in patients taking Vioxx compared to those taking a pain medication called naproxen. The Food and Drug Administration then asked Merck to add a warning to the drug's label.

But Merck said that the company had conducted its own regularly updated analyses of clinical trial data on Vioxx and had not determined there was a problem until 2004.

"Based on our own analyses, we did not see an increase in cardiovascular events with Vioxx compared to a placebo," Doug Watson, a cardiovascular epidemiologist at Merck, said in a phone interview Monday.

Requiring the kind of constant cumulative analyses for all drugs proposed in the Ross article would require an act of Congress, said Dr. Janet Woodcock, the director of the F.D.A.'s Center for Drug Evaluation and Research.

The F.D.A. has stepped up its safety measures since reports of heart problems with Vioxx first surfaced, Dr. Woodcock said. The agency has added staff members in all divisions to monitor drug safety, has strengthened its Office of Surveillance and Epidemiology and has instituted a postmarket safety tracking system for new drugs, she said. The agency also regularly conducts its own meta-analyses of drug safety, particularly when there is a signal of a health problem, Dr. Woodcock said.

Meanwhile, in 2007, Congress passed an amendment to federal drug law that has given the agency authority to require drug makers to put in place risk management programs for certain drugs and to conduct postmarket safety studies, she said. The amendment also gives the agency the power to order changes to drug labels to reflect new safety information and requires drug makers to make public the results of clinical trials.

But some critics said Congress should give the agency more power – and more resources – to provide more detailed drug safety information to doctors and consumers. More information would be helpful, these critics said, because the studies required to gain approval for a new drug are often too short in duration or too small to identify all serious side effects. Sometimes, problems associated with a drug may not become known until it is used over time by several hundreds of thousands of people, they said.

Dr. Woodcock said cumulative analyses of the type the Ross article proposes could be useful to check out hypotheses about particular safety problems associated with particular drugs.

But there are so many drugs on the market that it would probably be impossible, if not prohibitively expensive, to cumulatively track all of them, said Dr. Elliott M. Antman, a professor of medicine at the Harvard Medical School. Still, Dr. Antman said it would make sense for the agency to give conditional approval to certain new drugs, requiring drug makers to file cumulative analyses of safety and efficacy data several years later in order to obtain permanent approval.

[By Natasha Singer Published: November 23, 2009, adapted from]

WORD FILE

- **Blockbuster:** a book, a film or a product which is very good or successful.
- **Blueprint:** a plan for achieving something (technical); a pattern that all living cells contain, which decides how a person, animal or plant develops and what it looks like (*By changing the genetic blueprint of fruit, scientists can...*).

- **Evidence:** prova.
- **Injury claim:** richiesta di risarcimento per lesioni.
- **Litigation:** controversia legale.
- **Publicly:** pubblicamente.
- **Step up (to):** migliorare.
- **Track (to):** seguire le tracce (percorso).
- **Updated:** aggiornato.
- **Withdraw (to), withdrew, withdrawn:** ritirare.

Palliative Care
Palliative care is an approach that improves the quality of life of patients and their families facing the problem associated with life-threatening illness, through the prevention and relief of suffering by means of early identification and impeccable assessment and treatment of pain and other problems, physical, psychosocial and spiritual.
WHO (World Health Organization)

Exercise 5

Decide which statements are true (T) or false (F).

	T	F
1. Vioxx was a bestseller drug for the treatment of heart diseases.		
2. Vioxx was withdrawn from the market because of clinical studies proving its possibility of harms.		

3. There is a proposal for a drug monitoring consisting in a database which could be freely analyzed.
4. The use of a continuously updated model is proposed as a post market surveillance to avoid the risks of a treatment.
5. Dr Ross had been involved in the lawsuits against Merck as a consultant.
6. Merck declared disagreement about the methodology of the study's authors.
7. The FDA has stepped up a postmarket safety tracking system for new drugs.
8. The studies required to give approval to new drugs are considered, in some aspects, not suitable for the identification of all the side effects.
9. The cumulative tracking of all the drugs is considered prohibitively expensive.

Exercise 6

Give the Italian for.

1. This pain medication for arthritis became a blockbuster ....
2. A fuller picture of a drug's harms and benefits ....
3. The lead author of the study ....
4. For high risk drugs this could be a blueprint going forward ....
5. The new study proposes a continuously updated model ....
6. The Company voluntarly withdrew the drug within a week of learning that ....

Exercise 7

Read the text below and decide which answers best fit each gap.

FDA's Role in Assuring Safe and Effective Drugs

[A] .... the authority of the Federal Food, Drug, and Cosmetic Act and other laws, the Food and Drug Administration (FDA) [B] .... that new drugs developed by pharmaceutical companies are safe and effective and supported [C] .... rigorous scientific research. This typically [D] .... pharmaceutical companies to conduct extensive pre-clinical and clinical testing spanning 12 to 15 years and costing upwards of $800 million for [E] .... new drug. The FDA-approved drug label distills this mountain of data into a clear set of instructions that permits physicians [F] .... the drug product safely and effectively.

Pre-clinical Testing

Before a new drug can be tested in human volunteers (clinical testing), it [G] .... be shown to be reasonably safe in pre-clinical tests. Pre-clinical testing – [H] .... involves testing the drug product in animals – [I] .... an early warning regarding possible safety risks of a drug product. The FDA reviews the pre-clinical testing of a new drug and examines the company's proposed research plan before [L] .... trials in humans to begin.

Clinical Studies

Clinical studies – which involve testing a drug product in human volunteers – [M] .... and must follow the pre-set research plan approved by the FDA. Also, the FDA requires an Investigation-al Review Board (IRB) composed of community health care practitioners to review and approve all studies [N] .... human subjects. IRBs ensure that the risks to patients are minimized, that patients' rights are protected, and that informed consent and privacy are obtained. Once the clinical studies [O] ...., information gathered from the study is regularly submitted to the FDA for ongoing review. Controlled clinical studies are the only legal basis for the FDA to conclude that a new drug is safe and effective for use.

Drug Approval

After all clinical studies [P] ...., the FDA reviews the data and decides whether the drug can be placed on the market. To be considered for approval, the following information [Q] .... to FDA:

- documentation of the clinical test results;
- the drug's components;
- results of animal studies;
- how the drug [R] .... manufactured, processed, and packaged;
- drug samples;
- the proposed drug label with complete prescribing information.

Before [S] .... a drug, the FDA makes on-site visits to the investigators responsible for the clinical studies. The FDA approves the drug if the results of controlled clinical studies show effectiveness of the drug and that the product is safe [T] .... the conditions of use in the proposed labeling. Once a drug is approved, the FDA continues to monitor the safety and quality of the drug by, [U] .... other things, requiring drug manufacturers to comply with FDA's good manufacturing-practices requirements. The FDA also oversees the promotion and advertising of prescription drugs. Companies continue their responsibility [V] .... for safety and promptly reporting serious side effects of the drug to the FDA.

A	1 under	2 on	3 to ensure
B	1 ensures	2 ensuring	3 to ensure
C	1 from	2 by	3 over
D	1 requires	2 required	3 has required
E	1 all	2 several	3 each
F	1 use	2 using	3 to use
G	1 shall	2 has	3 must
H	1 whose	2 who	3 which
I	1 providing	2 provides	3 to provide
L	1 allowing	2 to allow	3 allowed
M	1 control	2 controlling	3 are controlled
N	1 to involve	2 involving	3 involved
O	1 are started	2 start	3 have started
P	1 have completed	2 are completed	3 have been completed
Q	1 must submit	2 have submitted	3 must be submitted
R	1 has	2 is	3 are
S	1 approving	2 to approve	3 having approved
T	1 above	2 by	3 under
U	1 between	2 within	3 among
V	1 to monitor	2 by monitoring	3 from monitoring

UNIT 5

FLU & VACCINES

SEASONAL FLU

Influenza (the flu) is a contagious respiratory illness caused by influenza viruses. It spreads from person-to-person and can cause mild to severe illness; and in some cases, can lead to death. In the United States, yearly outbreaks of seasonal flu usually happen during the fall through early spring. The best way to prevent the flu is by getting a flu vaccination each year.

All types of flu can cause fever, coughing and/or sore throat, runny or stuffy nose, headaches and/or body aches, chills, and fatigue.

Although flu viruses can cause illness in people of any age group, children are most likely to get sick because their immune systems aren't strong enough to fight off the infection. In addition to children, some groups are more likely to have complications from the seasonal flu. These include those age 65 and older people of any age who have chronic medical conditions (e.g. diabetes, asthma, congestive heart failure, lung disease). Complications from the flu can include bacterial pneumonia, ear or sinus infections, dehydration, and worsening of chronic medical conditions.

A flu pandemic occurs when a new influenza A virus emerges for which there is little or no immunity in the human population; the virus causes serious illness and spreads easily from person-to-person worldwide.

True influenza is an acute infectious disease caused by a member of the orthomyxovirus family: influenza virus A, B or, to a much lesser extent, influenza virus C. However, the term 'flu' is often used for any febrile respiratory illness with systemic symptoms that may be caused by a myriad of bacterial or viral agents as well as influenza viruses. Influenza outbreaks usually occur in the winter in temperate climates. In the United States, the flu season usually starts in October or November and is at its height from December to March. Every year in the United States, on average 5 to 20 percent of the population get the flu and more than 200,000 people are hospitalized from flu-related complications. Of these, about 36,000 people die from flu-related causes.

The virus is spread person to person via small particle aerosols (less then 10 μm diameter) that can get into the respiratory tract. The incubation period is short, about 18 to 72 hours.

Virus concentration in nasal and tracheal secrections remains high for 24 to 48 hours after symptoms start and may last longer in children. Titers are usually high and so there are enough infections virions in a small droplet to start a new infection. Influenza virus infects the epitelial cells of the respiratory tract. The cells die, in part due to the direct effects of the virus on the cell, and also possibly due to the effects of interferon. Cell death at later times may also result from the actions of cytotoxic T-cells. As a result, the efficiency of ciliary clearance is reduced, leading to impaired mucus excretion; thus there is reduced clearance of infectious agents from the respiratory tract.

Interferon may play a role by decreasing virus production. Many of the symptoms of uncomplicated influenza (muscle aches, fatigue, fever) are associated with the efficient induction of interferon. The cell mediated immune response is important in viral clearance as the antibody response is usually not significant until after virus has been cleared. Repair of the respiratory epithelium begins rapidly, but may take some time to complete.
A humoral antibody response is the main source of protection. IgG persists longer than IgA and so play a more important role in long term immunity.

Exercise 1

Complete according to the text.

1. Seasonal flu spreads from ....
2. It causes .... illness.
3. In some cases it can lead to ....
4. The outbreaks of seasonal flu .... happen ....
5. The best way to prevent it is ....
6. Some groups of people are more likely to have .... from ....
7. These groups include ....
8. A flu pandemic occurs ....
9. A virus causes .... and spreads ....

Pay attention

Flu ➢ a common illness that makes you feel very tired and weak. It causes a sore throat, cough and runny nose
Joe is still in bed with flu. Jane has got flu. I had flu last week. Flu virus/flu epidemic.
The word flu is **uncountable**.

e.g. ➢ means for example
from the latin "exempli gratia"

Exercise 2

Decide which statements are true (T) or false (F).

	T	F
1. Any febrile respiratory illness can be defined as "influenza".	■	■
2. Every year more than 200,000 people in the US get the flu.	■	■
3. Flu symptoms generally last longer in children.	■	■
4. The respiratory tract epithelial cells are those which are infected by the flu virus.	■	■
5. Cell death is mainly due to the effects of interferon.	■	■
6. The virus production is affected by interferon.	■	■
7. The antibody response generally works after the virus clearance.	■	■
8. In long term immunity IgG turns up to be more important than IgA.	■	■

SWINE INFLUENZA

Swine Influenza (swine flu) is a respiratory disease of pigs caused by type A influenza virus that regularly causes outbreaks of influenza in pigs. Swine flu viruses cause high levels of illness and low death rates in pigs. The classical swine flu virus (an influenza type A H1N1 virus) was first isolated from a pig in 1930.

Like all influenza viruses, swine flu viruses change constantly. Pigs can be infected by avian influenza and human influenza viruses as well as swine influenza viruses. When influenza viruses from different species infect pigs, the viruses can reassort (i.e. swap genes) and new viruses that are a mix of swine, human and/or avian influenza viruses can emerge. Over the years, different variations of swine flu viruses have emerged. At this time, there are four main influenza type A virus subtypes that have been isolated in pigs: H1N1, H1N2, H3N2, and H3N1. However, most of the recently isolated influenza viruses from pigs have been H1N1 viruses.

Swine flu viruses do not normally infect humans. However, sporadic human infections with swine flu have occurred. Most commonly, these cases occur in persons with direct exposure to pigs (e.g. children near pigs at a fair or workers in the swine industry).

In the past, CDC received reports of approximately one human swine influenza virus infection every one to two years in the US, but from December 2005 through February 2009, 12 cases of human infection with swine influenza have been reported.

The symptoms of swine flu in people are expected to be similar to the symptoms of regular human seasonal influenza and include fever, lethargy, lack of appetite and coughing. Some people with swine flu also have reported runny nose, sore throat, nausea, vomiting and diarrhea.

Influenza viruses can be directly transmitted from pigs to people and from people to pigs. Human infection with flu viruses from pigs are most likely to occur when people are in close proximity to infected pigs, such as in pig barns and livestock exhibits housing pigs at fairs. Human-to-human transmission of swine flu can also occur. This is thought to occur in the same way as seasonal flu occurs in people, which is mainly person-to-person transmission through coughing or sneezing of people infected with the influenza virus. People may become infected by touching something with flu viruses on it and then touching their mouth or nose.

To diagnose swine influenza A infection, a respiratory specimen would generally need to be collected within the first 4 to 5 days of illness (when an infected person is most likely to be shedding virus). Several different antiviral drugs are licensed for use in the US for the treatment of influenza, such as amantadine, rimantadine, oseltamivir and zanamivir. While most swine influenza viruses have been susceptible to all four drugs, the most recent swine influenza viruses isolated from humans are resistant to amantadine and rimantadine. At this time, CDC recommends the use of oseltamivir or zanamivir for the treatment and/or prevention of infection with swine influenza viruses.

The H1N1 swine flu viruses are antigenically very different from human H1N1 viruses and, therefore, vaccines for human seasonal flu can only provide a partial protection against swine H3N2, but not swine H1N1 virus.

Pandemia

According to the World Health Organization (WHO), a pandemic can start when three conditions have been met:

- **emergence of a disease new to a population;**
- **agents infect humans, causing serious illness; and**
- **agents spread easily and sustainably among humans.**

A disease or condition is not a pandemic merely because it is widespread or kills many people; it must also be infectious.

Exercise 3

Answer the following questions.

1. What is swine flu caused by?

....

....

2. Does it cause a high percentage of deaths in pigs?

....

....

3. Which are the symptoms of swine flu?

....

....

4. How does it occur that flu virus are transmitted from pigs to humans?

....

....

5. Name antiviral drugs that are licensed for the treatment of flu in the US.

....

....

Exercise 4

Complete according to the text.

1. To diagnose swine flu A infection, a respiratory specimen generally needs to ....

....

2. There are four main influenza type A virus subtypes that ....

....

3. Swine flu can be transmitted person to person in the same way as seasonal flu, which is mainly

....

4. Vaccines for human seasonal flu can only provide ....

....

TAMIFLU IN BRIEF

Tamiflu (oseltamivir), a prescription drug, is an oral antiviral treatment (not a vaccine!) for influenza, and belongs to a class of medicines called neuraminidase inhibitors (NAI). These medicines prevent the influenza virus from spreading inside the body and are designed to be active against all clinically relevant influenza virus strains. Tamiflu can be used both for prevention and treatment of influenza.

Neuraminidase is an enzyme that enables the virus to continue to infect host cells. When neuraminidase is inhibited, the virus is unable to exit the host cell and dies. Therefore the virus is not able to spread to and infect other cells in the body. In contrast to the older antivirals, the M2 inhibitors,

NAIs are effective against both influenza A and B viruses.

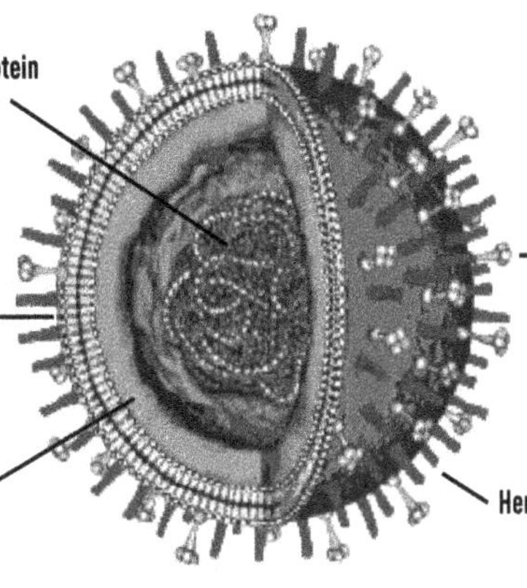

Tamiflu is proven to be effective in the treatment and for the prevention of influenza in adults and in children 1 year and older.

Tamiflu is given orally, as a convenient capsule and is systemically absorbed, meaning that it can reach key sites in the body where the virus multiplies. The dose for the adult treatment of influenza is a 75 mg capsule, taken twice daily for five days. One pack of Tamiflu contains a full treatment course of 102/110 capsules. Treatment must commence within 48 hours of the onset of symptoms for full efficacy. For post exposure prophylaxis in adults the dosage is one 75 mg capsule daily for 10 days and for seasonal prophylaxis the dose is one 75 mg capsule daily for up to 6 weeks.

In 1996 Roche acquired the worldwide rights to develop and market the drug from Gilead Sciences, Foster City, California.

Tamiflu was launched in North America (US and Canada) and Switzerland during 1999/2000. It was launched in all key European markets by 2002/2003.

Around 42 million patients have been treated to date with Tamiflu in about 80 countries worldwide including United States, Japan, Canada, Australia, the EU, Switzerland and Latin America.

Tamiflu is patent protected until 2016; the patent is owned by Gilead.

Tamiflu Efficacy

When administered according to its approved dosage (75 mg twice daily for 5 days), there is a reduction in the duration of influenza illness. Tamiflu also reduces the severity of symptoms and lower respiratory tracts infections, such as bronchitis, in otherwise healthy individuals.

In children Tamiflu reduces the duration of influenza illness and the severity of symptoms. There is also a reduction in incidence of associated otitis media as compared to standard care.

In adults Tamiflu is effective in protecting individual persons against influenza illness and is effective in preventing outbreaks in households. In children Tamiflu is effective in reducing the likelihood of febrile influenza in households with a positive index case. Tamiflu reduces the overall amount of virus and significantly reduces the amount of viral shedding in the body.

Active Immunization or Vaccination

The terms vaccination and vaccine derive from the work of Edward Jenner who, over 200 years ago, showed that inoculating people with material from skin lesions caused by cowpox (L. vaccinus, of cows) protected them from the highly contagious and frequently fatal disease smallpox.

Since Jenner's time, the term has been retained for any preparation of dead or weakened pathogens, or their products, that when introduced into the body, stimulates the production of protective antibodies or T cells without causing the disease. In molecular terms, the goal is to introduce harmless antigen(s) with epitopes that are also found on the pathogen.

Vaccination is also called active immunization because the immune system is stimulated to develop its own immunity against the pathogen. Passive immunity, in contrast, results from the injection of antibodies formed by another animal (e.g., horse, human) which provide immediate, but temporary, protection for the recipient.

Tamiflu Safety Data

Tamiflu has been used by several tens of million people worldwide since launch and has been found to have a favourable safety profile and is well tolerated. The majority of adverse events are gastrointestinal and self limiting and seldom lead to treatment discontinuation.

Exercise 5

Here are some of the most common vaccines. Can you get the Italian correspondent words?

1. Diphtheria. ....
2. Polio. ....
3. Pertussis. ....
4. Tetanus. ....
5. Hepatitis. ....
6. Measles. ....
7. Mumps. ....
8. Rubella. ....
9. Chickenpox. ....
10. Smallpox. ....
11. Thyphus. ....

WORD FILE

- **Adjuvant:** any substance that enhances the potency and effectiveness of an antigen.
- **Antigen:** any substance eliciting an immunologic response such as the production of antibody specific for that substance.
- **Dose:** a single portion or quantity of a therapeutic agent (medicine). *Dose sparing:* che permette di risparmiare sul dosaggio. *Low dose:* basso dosaggio.
- **Endemic:** found regularly in a particular place.
- **Epitope:** The part of the macromolecule that is recognized by the immune system.
- **Lead (to), led, led:** guide or conduct. *Leader:* person who leads. *Leading:* principale. *Lead-in:* introduzione di un argomento. *Lead (n.):* piombo; guinzaglio.
- **Stockpile:** a large supply of things that is kept ready for use in the future.
- **Strain:** a group of organisms possessing a common characteristic distinguishing them from others within the same species.
- **Titer:** an expression of the strength of a volumetric solution. Amount of the quantity of a substance.
- **Trial:** the act of trying or testing.

- **Arise (to), arose, arisen:** sorgere, alzarsi.
- **Closely:** da vicino. *Close to:* vicino a.
- **Concern:** interesse, preoccupazione, coinvolgimento. *Ongoing concern:* crescente preoccupazione.

- **Deadliness:** mortalità, letalità.
- **Despite:** malgrado, a dispetto di.
- **Do (to), did, done:** fare.
- **Engage (to):** impegnare, impegnarsi.
- **Enhance (to):** intensificare, aumentare, valorizzare.
- **Facilities (pl):** impianto, struttura, installazione.
- **Find (to), found, found:** trovare.
- **Furthermore:** inoltre.
- **Health:** salute, sanità.
- **Hinder (to):** impedire.
- **Make (to), made, made:** fare.
- **Outbreak:** focolaio, esplosione.
- **To outbreak/to break, broke, broken:** rompere.
- **Over time:** tempo supplementare, oltre il tempo fissato.
- **Pattern:** modello, schema (*Patterns of infection*).
- **Take (to), took, taken:** prendere. *Take place:* aver luogo.
- **Win (to), won, won:** vincere.

Pay attention

150 million doses ➢ millions of doses.
Two hundred dollars ➢ hundreds of dollars.
Five thousand people ➢ thousands of people.

Exercise 6

Fill in the blanks using words from the box. (Pay attention! The given words are more than what you need.)

• any • for use • may • clinicians • older • sick • severe • be used • to prevent
• will • learn • would • can • recommends • started • avoid • prevent
• complications • starts • range • milder • sensitive • so far
• health care professional • benefit • infection • pills • antiviral
• hay fever • person • detected • have

Antiviral Drugs

Antiviral drugs are prescription medicines (..................., liquid or an inhaler) with activity against influenza viruses, including swine influenza viruses. Antiviral drugs can be used to treat swine flu or to prevent .... with swine flu viruses. These medications must be prescribed by a .... Influenza antiviral drugs only work against influenza viruses –f they will not help treat or .... symptoms caused by infection from other viruses that can cause symptoms similar to the flu.

There are four influenza antiviral drugs approved .... in the United States (oseltamivir, zanamivir, amantadine and rimantadine). The swine influenza A (H1N1) viruses that have been .... in humans in the United States and Mexico are resistant to amantadine and rimantadine so these drugs will not work against these swine influenza viruses. Laboratory testing on these swine influenza A (H1N1) viruses .... indicate that they are .... to oseltamivir and zanamivir.

Benefits of Antiviral Drugs

- Treatment: If you get ...., antiviral drugs can make your illness .... and make you feel better faster. They may also prevent serious influenza .... For treatment, antiviral drugs work best if started as soon after getting sick as possible, and might not work if .... more than 48 hours after illness ....
- Prevention: Influenza antiviral drugs also can be used to prevent influenza when they are given to a person who is not ill, but who has been or .... be near a person with swine influenza. When used to prevent the flu, antiviral drugs are about 70% to 90% effective. When used for prevention, the number of days that they should .... will vary depending on a person's particular situation.

CDC Recommendation

CDC .... the use of oseltamivir or zanamivir for the treatment and/or prevention of infection with swine influenza viruses.

Oseltamivir (brand name Tamiflu®) is approved to both treat and prevent influenza A and B virus infection in people one year of age and ....

Zanamivir (brand name Relenza®) is approved to treat influenza A and B virus infection in people 7 years and older and .... influenza A and B virus infection in people 5 years and older.

Recommendations for using antiviral drugs for treatment or prevention of swine influenza .... change as we .... more about this new virus.

.... should consider treating .... person with confirmed or suspected swine influenza with an antiviral drug.

Visit: www.cdc.gov/swineflu/recommendations.htm for specific recommendations.

Links to non-federal organizations are provided solely as a service to our users. These links do not constitute an endorsement of these organizations or their programs by CDC or the federal government, and none should be inferred. CDC is not responsible for the content of the individual organization Web pages found at these links.

CDC The Centers for Disease Control and Prevention, the US agency charged with tracking and investigating public health trends. The stated mission of the CDC is "To promote health and quality of life by preventing and controlling disease, injury, and disability." The CDC is a part of the US Public Health Services (PHS) under the Department of Health and Human Services (HHS).

Exercise 7

Read this article and decide which statements are true (T) or false (F).

For decades, vaccines have provided effective protection from influenza for Americans. While they have traditionally been produced in chicken eggs, a new technology-cell-based vaccine production could save hundreds of thousands of lives in the event of an outbreak of pandemic influenza, or some other infectious disease.

The new approach would use mammalian cells (kidney cells are often used) to grow the influenza viruses. Cell-based vaccine production could more easily meet "surge capacity needs" because cells could be frozen and stored in advance of an epidemic or developed rapidly in response to an epidemic. Cell-based vaccine production dramatically reduces the possibility for contamination and promises to be more reliable, flexible, and expandable than egg-based methods.

In place of eggs, cell-based vaccine production utilizes laboratory-grown cell lines that are capable of hosting a growing virus. The virus is injected into the cells where it multiplies. The cells' outer walls are removed, harvested, purified, and inactivated. A vaccine can be produced in a matter of weeks. Polio vaccine is currently produced using the cell-based method.

While both methods could produce an equally effective vaccine, egg-based production is physically limited by the availability of specialized eggs and alone may not be able to meet the accelerated demands of a global influenza pandemic. Cell-based vaccines offer the potential to increase production surge capacity and save lives:

- In order to produce 300 million doses of vaccine, egg-based production would require some 900 million eggs. In the case of an avian flu pandemic, egg-producing flocks could decline, jeopardizing vaccine production capabilities.
- While eggs are perishable, cell lines can be safely kept frozen indefinitely, increasing the capability to rapidly produce vaccines if an influenza pandemic were to occur.
- Vaccine manufacturers are able to bypass the steps needed to adapt the virus strains to grow in eggs.
- People allergic to eggs cannot receive vaccines produced from chicken eggs, but can be immunized with a cell-based vaccine.

In March 2005, the Department of Health and Human Services issued a five-year contract to Sanofi-Pasteur for $97.1 million to develop cell-based influenza vaccine technology and conduct clinical trials, with the goal of obtaining an FDA license for this vaccine. Under this advanced development contract, the company has committed to develop a plan to establish a US cell-based influenza vaccine manufacturing facility, capable of producing at least 300 million doses of a pandemic influenza vaccine over a one year period.

	T	F
1. Egg-based vaccine production is unable to meet requirements in case of pandemic influenza.	▢	▢
2. Egg based methods allow a quick production of vaccines.	▢	▢
3. Kidney cells are generally used in cell-based vaccine production.	▢	▢
4. Cell based production is now preferred because of its possibility of easy storage.	▢	▢
5. The two methods aren't equally effective against flu owing to cell freezing possibility.	▢	▢
6. Allergic people can't be immunized by egg-based vaccines.	▢	▢
7. Agreements aiming to ensure a mass production of vaccine were carried out in 2005.	▢	▢
8. Polio vaccine is produced through the egg-based methods.	▢	▢

Exercise 8

Translate the following Italian phares using compund nouns.

1. Ceppi del virus dell'influenza. ....
2. La prevenzione dell'influenza. ....
3. La cura dell'influenza per adulti. ....
4. Lesioni della pelle. ....
5. Nuova tecnologia per la produzione di vaccini. ....

Exercise 9

Choose the correct word for each space.

Cell culture-derived influenza vaccine technology is [A] .... production process for the [B] .... of flu vaccine on the [C] .... of cell cultures. Cell culture-derived influenza vaccines (commonly [D] .... as "flu cell culture"vaccines) use cell cultures [E] .... than chicken eggs for antigen production. Current egg-derived vaccines production requires [F] .... nine months, and this lead time can hinder the response to unanticipated demands such as the [G] .... of pandemic strains, production failures and [H] .... influenza virus strain changes. In contrast, flu cell culture production [I] .... flexible, faster start-up of vaccine manufacturing, [L] .... a particularly important advantage in the [M] .... of an influenza pandemic. Novartis is a [N] .... in cell culture-derive influenza vaccine development, with advances in its US and EU trials [O] .... announced in October 2005.

A	1 an innovative	2 a proved	3 a basic	4 an old
B	1 manufacturing	2 working	3 discovering	4 making
C	1 links	2 based	3 basis	4 studies
D	1 called	2 referred to	3 underlined	4 linked
E	1 even	2 as	3 rather	4 after
F	1 most	2 up to	3 few than	4 less
G	1 protection	2 response	3 discovery	4 adjuvant
H	1 seasonal	2 human	3 current	4 recent
I	1 tries	2 stops	3 works	4 enables
L	1 preventing	2 arranging	3 providing	4 including
M	1 basis	2 fact	3 reason	4 event
N	1 leader	2 company	3 authority	4 institute
O	1 as	2 when	3 for	4 like

UNIT 6

DRUG DEVELOPMENT

PHARMACOLOGY

Pharmacology is one of the cornerstones of the drug discovery process. The medicinal chemist may create the candidate compound, but the pharmacologist is the one who tests it for physiologic activity. A promising compound is investigated by many other scientists – toxicologists, microbiologists, clinicians – but only after the pharmacologist has documented a potential therapeutic effect. This article briefly presents the historical development of pharmacology and some of the basic methods used.

Etymologically, pharmacology is the science of drugs (Greek pharmakos, medicine or drug; and logos, study). In actual use, however, its meaning is limited to the study of the actions of drugs. Pharmacology has been defined as "an experimental science which has for its purpose the study of changes brought about in living organisms by chemically acting substances (with the exception of foods), whether used for therapeutic purposes or not."

Pharmacology studies the effects of drugs and how they exert their effects. There is a distinction between what a drug does and how it acts. Thus, amoxicillin cures a strep throat, and cimetidine promotes the healing of duodenal ulcers. Pharmacology asks "How"? Amoxicillin inhibits the synthesis of cell wall mucopeptide by the bacteria that cause the infection, and cimetidine inhibits gastric acid secretion by its antagonist action on histamine H2 receptors.

The main tasks of pharmacologists, in the search for and development of new medicines, are

- screening for desired activity
- determining mode of action, and
- quantifying drug activity when chemical methods are not available.

Basic Techniques

Experimental pharmacology uses animals in various ways. Intact animals are essential for the acute, subacute, and chronic toxicity tests that a new drug substance must undergo, and for important special tests such as teratology and carcinogenicity. Pharmacology per se tends to use excised (isolated) organs or tissues and animals that are surgically prepared in various ways to aid in the detection and study of target activities.

Early in the development of pharmacologic techniques, it was found that an isolated organ or tissue remained functional for several hours in a bath containing a physiologic solution of salts through which oxygen was bubbled. Henrick Magnus (1802-1870) first applied this method to a strip of small intestine, Jean-François Heymans (1904) worked with the mammalian heart, and Claude Bernard experimented with isolated nerve–muscle preparations.

The organ or tissue is so suspended that the contraction or relaxation of the muscle is mechanically transmitted to a stylet. The stylet writes on a drum covered with smoked paper rotated by clockwork at a constant speed. This device, called a kymograph, graphically records motion or pressure. The effects of drug substances added to the bath can thus be visualized. The kymograph is a relatively crude device. In modern laboratories, organ and tissue movements are transmitted by force transducers to polygraph machines, which produce similar tracings. Or the polygraph is replaced by computerized equipment that issues a digital record.

Pay attention

Equipment ➢ sempre singolare.

Rational Design

Screening of candidate compounds and mode-of-action studies may focus on specific tissues, organs, or systems or on actions, such as antihistaminic or anticonvulsant. As knowledge of human biochemistry and molecular biology advances, pharmacology zeroes in more often on enzymatic action and receptors.

Knowledge of cell receptors is now on the cutting edge of pharmacology and drug discovery. The concept was first proposed about a hundred years ago by Paul Ehrlich, the great bacteriologist and chemist who synthesized salvarsan (also known as "606") for the treatment of syphilis. On the basis of his research on bacterial toxins, Ehrlich postulated that the body's cells possess a great many "receptors" by which they combine with the food substances in the body fluids. He theorized that the metabolic products of certain bacteria combine with the receptors of some cells, thus injuring the cells. Ehrlich visualized receptors as unsatisfied chemical side chains. This is not far from the modern idea of receptors as domains in enzymes or other proteins, with which drugs of appropriate structure can combine.

WORD FILE

- **Biochemistry:** the scientific study of the chemistry of living things. *Biochemical* (adj.).
- **Muscle:** one of the pieces of flesh inside your body that you use in order to move, and that connect your bones together.
- **Receptor:** protein present in cells that specifically recognize molecules (agonists) that cause cells to respond in particular ways.
- **Toxin:** a poisonous substance, especially one that is produced by bacteria and causes a particular disease.

- **Be at the cutting edge (to):** essere all'avanguardia.
- **Clockwork:** meccanismo a molla.
- **Exert (to):** esercitare, esplicare.
- **Injure (to):** ferire.
- **Stylet:** stiletto, pennino.
- **Undergo (to):** subire, essere sottoposto a.

Exercise 1

Answer the following questions.

1. What is the role of the pharmacologist?

 ....

2. What's the meaning of pharmacology?

 ....

3. Which are the main tasks pharmacologists are supposed to face?

 ....

4. Where does the knowledge of cell receptors lead?

 ....

5. What does amoxicillin cure and what are its effects?

 ....

6. How does cimetidine act in treating duodenal ulcers?

 ....

Exercise 2

Give the Italian for.

1. On the cutting edge of pharmacology ....
2. Surgically prepared ....
3. A drum covered with a smoked paper ....
4. This device graphically records ....
5. Unsatisfied chemical side chains ....
6. It is replaced by computerized equipment ....

Exercise 3

Read the following text carefully and answer the questions.

PUBLIC LECTURE: DEFEATING THE ENEMY WITHIN - CANCER DRUG DESIGN FOR THE NEW MILLENNIUM

Cancer is probably the most important disease of modern western society, and, despite many advances, much remains to be done in the development of new treatments. The public lecture will explain what cancer is, how cancerous cells differ from normal cells and how these differences can be exploited for the development of more effective drugs. The lecture will take place on Wednesday 7 May from 5.15-6.15pm on the Claverton campus.

The lecture will be given by Dr Matthew Lloyd in the Department of Pharmacy & Pharmacology. Dr Lloyd is part of a team of researchers at Bath that were awarded more than £450,000 by Cancer Research UK to investigate a new way of preventing the division and growth of tumour cells. During the talk, a donation will be made by the Pharmacy Students Association (PSA) to Sabrina Sallis, the local Cancer Research UK fundraising officer. The association raises money for charity each year and chose to donate to Cancer Research UK on the basis of the department's recent research success.

Sophie Blow from the PSA said: "Cancer is a disease affecting 1 in 3 people and so most students in the department know someone who has suffered from the disease and therefore were very supportive of the committee in this donation."
Research by Dr Lloyd and his colleagues targets a family of enzymes – types of worker molecules – that appear to be involved in controlling cell growth. Studies have shown that increased levels of these enzymes, known as sirtuins, are found in tumours from a range of different cancer types.
This suggests that, by finding a way of preventing these enzymes from working, it may be possible to halt the progression of cancer by stopping tumour cells from dividing and growing.
Dr Mike Threadgill, who is leading the research, said: "The work funded by Cancer Research UK will build on a long history of successful anti-cancer work at the University of Bath. Colleagues already have a range of treatments currently in early stage clinical trials for hormone-dependent breast cancers. If successful, we would hope that by the end of this project we might be in a position to begin developing the compounds for clinical trials."
Dr Lloyd graduated with DPhil (PhD) in Chemistry & Biochemistry from the University of Oxford in 1992. Following post-doctoral experience at Brown University, USA and the University of Oxford, he joined the Department of Pharmacy & Pharmacology in 2002.
Admission is free, just turn up on the night. Free parking is available in the West car park. The presentation will take place in lecture theatre 8 West, 1.1 on the Claverton campus, University of Bath.
The University of Bath is one of the UK's leading universities, with an international reputation for quality research and teaching. In 15 subject areas the University of Bath is rated in the top ten in the country. View a full list of the University's press releases: www.bath.ac.uk/news/releases

[Press Release, 01 May 20..]

1. Who is the lecturer?

   ....

   ....

2. When is the lecture supposed to take place?

   ....

   ....

3. Who is Sabrina Sallis?

   ....

   ....

4. Does the PSA give money to the Cancer Research every year?

   ....

   ....

5. Why do PSA students felt supportive towards cancer diseases?

   ....

   ....

6. What are "sirtuins"?

   ....

   ....

7. Who is the leader of the research team?

   ....

   ....

Pay attention

Pay attention to the different use of **to say** and **to tell**.

To say, said, said ➢ dire.
Si usa:
– nel discorso indiretto quando non è espressa la persona a cui si parla (complemento di termine)
He said he was too tired to go out.
– nel discorso diretto, con o senza il complemento di termine, in questo caso preceduto da "to"
The nurse said " no more patients this afternoon".
The teacher said to us "Don't buy that anthology".

To tell, told, told ➢ dire.
Si usa:
– nel discorso indiretto quando è espresso il complemento di termine
Tell Joe I'm here. Lucy told me she wanted to leave by plane.
– nelle espressioni: *to tell the truth, to tell lies, to tell the time*

BIOLOGICAL DRUGS

Biological drugs include antibodies, interleukins, and vaccines, or any substance that is made from a living organism or its products and is used in the prevention, diagnosis, or treatment of diseases.
Biological drugs are also called biologic agents and biological agents.
These drugs are substances found in the immune system, such as antibodies and cytokines, but as drugs they are produced in a laboratory.
Biologic drugs include:

- Interferons (IFNs). Interferons are part of the immune system that belong to a class of substances called cytokines. Interferons are usually associated with viral infections, although they are also produced in response to bacteria and other foreign invaders.
- Interleukins (ILs). Interleukins are also cytokines. These chemicals are produced by a variety of cells in the immune system to regulate and mediate the white blood cells.
- Monoclonal antibodies (MOABs). Natural antibodies are proteins that fight off infections. Monoclonal antibodies are created artificially and can be targeted against specific cells or agents.
- Colony-stimulating factors (CSFs). Sometimes called hematopoietic growth factors, these drugs stimulate bone marrow stem cells to divide and develop into white blood cells, red blood cells and platelets.

Most of the biological drugs used by doctors today are monoclonal antibodies. Antibodies are a normal part of everyone's immune system. These antibodies help the body fight disease every day. Monoclonal antibodies on the other hand have been specially changed so that they can treat a specific disease. These are special in that when they are given to a person, they are able to find the specific area in the body which needs drug treatment. For example monoclonal antibodies are able to specially search and find cancer cells in the body and treat them only. These antibodies find diseased cells so well that they make it possible for patients to have safe and effective treatments with fewer side effects. Monoclonal antibodies do not pass though the body like normal medicines. That means that there is often less chance of side effects in other areas of the body not being treated. Nevertheless, as with any drug there are side effects. Most of the side effects are usually limited to mild to moderate, but sometimes biological drugs have rare side effects that can be severe and life-threatening.

The new treatments offer less discomfort and much better outcomes. For example, patients with rheumatoid arthritis being treated with the biological drug called Humira® can avoid the side effects such as sores in the mouth, nausea and vomiting which were common with older treatments. Humira® has a shorter treatment time and a longer time between remissions. The most common side effects of Humira® are injection site reaction, headaches and rash. However patients taking Humira® can also have serious but rare reactions such as infections, cancer and neurological reactions.

In 2008 there were only eighteen FDA-approved biological drugs on the market. These drugs are being used to treat such diseases as rheumatoid arthritis, irritable bowel syndrome and asthma. They are also being used to treat cancers such as B-cell lymphoma.

One of the biggest concerns of consumers when it comes to healthcare is cost. Biological drugs are currently more costly but will become cheaper in the future as they are made in larger quantities. The recognition of the potential benefits of these drugs has put them on the fast track for FDA approval. The development of biological drugs is growing so fast that most of these medicines have gained approval only within the last ten years. With the largest part of our population about to retire, placing more and more strain on the healthcare system, biological drugs may offer a solution.

Alfred Nobel (1833-1896) was born in Stockholm, Sweden, on October 21, 1833. Alfred Nobel's greatness lay in his ability to combine the penetrating mind of the scientist and inventor (in 1867 he patented the dynamite, a stable mix of nitroglycerin adsorbed into diatomaceous earth or kieselgur) with the forward-looking dynamism of the industrialist that founded more than 90 plants in 20 different countries. Nobel was fluent in several languages, and wrote poetry and drama. Nobel was also very interested in social and peace-related issues, and held views that were considered radical during his time. The Nobel Prizes became an extension and a fulfillment of his lifetime interests.

WORD FILE

- **Bacteria:** bacterium pl. very small living things, some of which cause illness or disease.
- **Bowel:** the system of tubes inside your body where food is made into solid waste material and through which it passes out of your body.
- **Interferon:** a chemical substance that is produced by your body to fight against viruses that cause disease.
- **Marrow:** the soft fatty substance in the hollow centre of bones (*A bone marrow transplant*).
- **Platelet:** one of the very small flat round cells in your blood that help it become solid when you bleed, so that you stop bleeding.
- **Rash:** a lot of red spots on someone's skin, caused by an illness.
- **Remission:** a period when a serious illness improves for a time.
- **Sore:** a painful, often red, place on your body caused by a wound or infection.

- **Retire (to):** andare in pensione.
- **Strain:** sforzo, tensione. Ceppo, origine.
- **Mild:** mite, lieve, blando.
- **Costly:** costoso.
- **Concern:** interesse, preoccupazione.
- **Nevertheless:** tuttavia.

Exercise 4

Fill in the table.

Drug	Effects
IFNs	
ILs	
MOABs	
CFSs	

Exercise 5

Complete according to the text.

1. Cost is one of the big ....
2. Biological drugs will become .... in the future because ....
3. Antibodies are .... and help ....
4. Rare and severe side effects can be caused ....
5. In the last ten years many biological medicines have ....

Exercise 6

Answer the following questions.

1. What is Humira?

   ....

   ....

2. For which treatment is it used?

   ....

   ....

3. Does it cause severe side effects?

   ....

   ....

4. Which are the main features of monoclonal drugs?

   ....

   ....

UNIT 7

ALLERGIES

HOW TO FIGHT ALLERGIES

Some allergens are simply impossible to avoid. You cannot live a normal life and completely avoid pollen, dust mites, mold spores, and certain other common triggers of allergic reactions. Many allergy sufferers use medications such as antihistamines and steroid nasal sprays to suppress their symptoms, and these medications are very effective in most. For people with very severe symptoms, and those who cannot take allergy medications, immunotherapy is an alternative.

Immunotherapy is the name for a treatment used by allergy specialists (allergists) to reduce sensitivity to allergens. This therapy is particularly useful for people with allergic rhinitis (sometimes called hay fever). Immunotherapy involves a series of injections (shots) given regularly for several years. In the past, this was called a serum, but this is an incorrect name. Most allergists now call this mixture an allergy extract. The first shots contain very tiny amounts of the antigen or antigens to which you are allergic. With progressively increasing dosages over time, your body will adjust to the antigen and become less sensitive to it. This process is called desensitization.

Immunotherapy is the only available treatment that can modify the natural course of the allergic disease. This means that a 3-to 5-year regimen of injections may result in long-term benefits that extend well beyond the completion of the regimen. Immunotherapy does not work for everyone and is only partly effective in some people, but it offers allergy sufferers the chance of eventually stopping medication or reducing the amount they have to take.

How Do the Shots Work?

Immunotherapy does not treat symptoms; it treats the immune system, the source of all allergic reactions. Although the exact details of how allergy shots work is unknown, we do know the general way they affect the immune system.

An allergic reaction occurs when the body is exposed to an external substance (the antigen) that the immune system interprets as a foreign invader. In allergic individuals, the immune system then makes an unusual (allergic) response that harms the body.

- The white blood cells produce an antibody to the antigen called immunoglobulin E, or IgE. This is called sensitization.
- When the antibody comes in contact with the antigen, it promotes the release of certain chemicals called mediators into affected tissues. Histamine is an example of a mediator.
- It is the effects of mediators on organs and cells that cause the symptoms of allergic reactions.
- This overreaction to a harmless substance is often called a hypersensitivity reaction.

Allergy shots desensitize you by turning down this immune response to the antigen. As a result of immunotherapy, the white blood cells no longer respond as strongly to the antigen, and less production of the immunoglobulin E antibody to this antigen occurs. So, when you are exposed to this antigen, less severe allergic reactions occur in affected areas like the eyes, nasal mucosal surfaces, and the bronchial airways.

Non Prescription Drug or Over the Counter (OTC)
An OTC is a pharmaceutical product, drug, or medicinal specialty whose dispensing or administration does not require medical authorization, and it can be used by the consumers under its own initiative and responsibility to prevent, relieve or to treat symptoms or mild diseases and that its use, in the form, conditions and authorized dosages are safe for the consumer.

Alavert, Claritin, Claritin RediTabs (rapidly disintegrating), Claritin-D, and Claritin-D 12-hour are examples of the brand names. Loratadine is the generic name. Loratadine is an antihistamine used to treat hay fever and allergies.

Why Is Loratadine Used?

Loratadine is a nonprescription (over-the-counter) antihistamine. It is a second-generation antihistamine and selectively inhibits binding of histamine to type 1 histamine receptors. Antihistamines compete with histamine for histamine receptor sites. By occupying the histamine receptor sites, they prevent histamine from its actions.

Loratadine is indicated for adults and children 2 years or older for temporary relief of symptoms caused by hay fever and allergies (runny nose, sneezing, itchy/watery eyes, scratchy nose or throat). It is available in a variety of forms, including tablets, oral disintegrating tablets, and syrup.

WORD FILE

- **Antibody:** a substance produced by your body to fight disease.
- **Antigen:** a substance that makes the body produce antibodies.
- **Desensitize (to):** to make someone react less strongly to something by making them become used to it (*Desensitize somebody to something*).
- **Dust:** dry powder consisting of extremely small bits of dirt that is in buildings on furniture, floors etc if they are not kept clean. Dry powder consisting of extremely small bits of earth or sand. Powder consisting of extremely small bits of a particular substance.
- **Hay fever:** medical condition, like a bad cold that is caused by breathing in pollen (dust from plants).
- **Histamine:** a chemical substance produced by your body during an allergic reaction.
- **Immune system:** the system by which your body protects itself against disease.
- **Mite:** a very small creature that lives in carpets, plants etc.
- **Mould (UK) Mold (US):** a soft green, grey, or black substance that grows on food which has been kept too long, and on objects that are in warm, wet air.
- **Pollen:** a fine powder produced by flowers, which is carried by the wind or by insects to other flowers of the same type, making them produce seeds.
- **Spore:** a cell like a seed that is produced by some plants such as mushrooms and can develop into a new plant.
- **Steroid:** a chemical that the body produces naturally or that can be made as a drug to treat illness and injuries. Steroids are sometimes used illegally by people doing sports to improve their performance.

Exercise 1

Give a list of the uncountable nouns you can find in the previous word file.

....

....

....

....

Exercise 2

Give the Italian for:

1. Runny nose ....
2. Watery eyes ....
3. Scratchy nose ....
4. Itchy eyes ....
5. Sneezing ....
6. Oral disintegrating tablets ....

Exercise 3

Decide which statements are true (T) or false (F).

	T	F
1. Allergens are known to be impossible to avoid.	☐	☐
2. Immunotherapy reduces sensitivity to allergens.	☐	☐
3. "Allergy extract" is the name presently given to a series of injections given to reduce sensitivity to allergens.	☐	☐
4. Antihistamines are an effective treatment in case of hay fever.	☐	☐
5. Histamine is an antibody produced by white blood cells.	☐	☐
6. The immune response can be turned down thanks to allergy shots.	☐	☐

ANTIHISTAMINES

Antihistamines are a structurally diverse group of drugs sharing the ability to block the H1 histamine receptor. Histamine causes bronchoconstriction, increases bowel peristalsis, is a vasodilator, and increases vascular permeability. These are all features of allergic reactions and the major use for these drugs is in the symptomatic relief of allergic conditions. These drugs also have antagonist properties at muscarinic and dopaminergic receptors. These properties may well be responsible for their decongestant and antiemetic actions.

Antihistamines that do not penetrate the CNS, such as loratadine and acrivastine, are less sedative than those that do.

Prescribed for

- Symptomatic treatment of allergic conditions (hay fever, urticaria);
- treatment of anaphylaxis and angio-oedema;
- prophylaxis against motion sickness;
- symptom relief for vertigo and Meniere's disease.

Cinnarizine has been used as a treatment for peripheral vascular disease because of its calcium channel blocking properties, but it is not recommended for this use.

Safety and Efficacy

- Antihistamines have antimuscarinic actions; avoid using them in patients with prostatic hyperplasia, closed-angle glaucoma, or pyloroduodenal obstruction;
- these drugs are probably safe in pregnancy, but their routine use is not recommended.

Avoid antihistamines in patients with severe hepatic insufficiency; the sedative action may precipitate coma.

- Most of these drugs do not require dosage reduction in renal insufficiency, but in the case of cetirizine it is recommanded to halve the dose.
- These drugs are principally used for symptomatic relief; always ensure that you have a clear idea of the diagnosis that is responsible for the symptoms. Reconsider the diagnosis if the patient does not improve.
- Warn the patient about the sedative effects of these drugs (including those that are less sedative). Those with a long duration of action may have a considerable hangover effect.

[*Oxford Handbook of Clinical Pharmacy*, adapted from]

WORD FILE

- **Anaphylaxis:** a state of immediate hypersensitivity following exposure to a foreign protein, drug etc. The clinical manifestation of such a state.
- **Antiemetic:** preventing nausea and vomiting (ag.). An agent preventing nausea and vomiting (n.).
- **Bowel:** the system of tubes inside your body where food is changed into solid waste material and through which it passes out of your body.
- **Cough:** the action or sound made when you cough (countable). A medical condition that makes you cough a lot (uncountable).
- **Diagnosis:** the process of discovering exactly what is wrong with someone or something by a close exam.
- **Itch:** an uncomfortable feeling on your skin that makes you want to rub it with your nails.
- **Pregnant:** if a woman or a female animal is pregnant she has an unborn baby growing inside her body (pregnancy).
- **Receptor:** protein present in cells that specifically recognize molecules (agonists) that cause the cells to respond in particular ways.
- **Sedation:** the use of drugs to make someone calm or go to sleep. Sedative.
- **Symptomatic:** showing that someone has a particular illness.

- **Effective:** efficace, efficiente, opertivo.
- **Ensure (to):** assicurare.
- **Halve (to):** dividere a metà.
- **Harmful:** nocivo, dannoso.
- **Hives:** orticaria.
- **Improve (to):** migliorare.
- **Proprietary remedies:** specialità protette da brevetto.
- **Relief:** sollievo, conforto.
- **Underlie (to):** essere al di sotto di.

Exercise 4

Decide which statements are true (T) or false (F).

		T	F
1.	Histamine is a vasodilatator.	■	■
2.	Antihistamines such as loratadine and acrivastine are the most sedative ones.	■	■
3.	Antihistamines are not recommended to pregnant women.	■	■
4.	Antihistamines are more effective than topical corticosteroid.	■	■
5.	It's better to halve the dose of cetirizine in case of renal insufficiency.	■	■
6.	Antihistamines have the power to block the H1 histamine receptor.	■	■
7.	Antihistamines can be used in case of patients with hepatic insufficiency.	■	■
8.	The topical use of antihistamines can induce contact sensitivity.	■	■
9.	"Non sedative" antihistamines are safe for people who drive.	■	■
10.	The sedative effect of antihistamines is useful in case of cough.	■	■
11.	Patients with Menière disease can get relief from antihistamines.	■	■

Exercise 5

Fill in the blanks with words from the box.

• sensitive • histamine • symptoms • chemicals • to be carried • involves • range
• months • hay fever • mid spring • spores • asthma • reaction • oak • affects • available
• suffers • childhood • cells • air-borne pollen • breathed in • an allergic reaction • allergy

Hay fever: a seasonal inconvenience

Hay fever may be a massive inconvenience to its ...., but the good news is that there are many different medicines .... to take away the discomfort.

During the spring and summer .... of most countries in the northern hemisphere, many people suffer an allergic .... to air-borne pollen and fungal .... that can disrupt their lives quite significantly. This condition is known as seasonal allergic rhinitis, but is more commonly called ....

In the UK hay fever .... about 20% of the population and often develops in .... or during the teenage years. People with allergies and other conditions such as .... are sometimes likely to suffer from hay fever too.

Some research has also shown that people become less .... to pollen as they get older, so it may disappear completely once a person reaches their mid forties.

Hay fever is caused by an .... to different types of an .... and, to a lesser extent, fungal spores.

Pollen is produced from a .... of plants including trees, grasses and weeds. The pollen from these types of plants is tiny and carried by the wind, which is why they are easily. ....

Pollen that is carried by insects is too large .... by the wind and therefore rarely causes hay fever.

The hay fever season usually starts in .... with tree pollen such as birch and .... reaching a peak in the late spring. As the summer continues, grass pollens become more problematic and by the autumn, weed pollen and fungal spores are the main culprits.

Once breathed in, the pollen sets off .... that causes the symptoms of hay fever that many of us know all too well. This allergic reaction .... the production of antibodies that attach themselves to special blood cells called mast cells, which produce the chemical, ..., as well causing the release of other chemicals from other types of .... It is this histamine that causes the acute .... of hay fever, while the other .... can enhance and prolong the symptoms.

WORD FILE

- **Air-borne pollen:** polline a trasmissione aerea (*Air-borne-infection*).
- **Birch:** betulla.
- **Culprit:** responsabile, colpevole.
- **Drowsiness:** sonnolenza.
- **Fungal spores:** spore fungine.
- **Mast cell:** mastcellula.
- **Oak:** quercia.
- **Runny (ag.):** liquefatto, che cola.
- **Sneeze (to):** starnutire.
- **Staff:** personale.
- **Stuff:** roba, materiale.
- **Stuff (to):** imbottire, riempire.
- **Stuffy nose:** naso chiuso.
- **To rid of, to get rid of:** liberarsi di.
- **Weeds:** erbacce.
- **Wheeze (to):** ansimare.

Exercise 6

Fill in the blanks with words from the box.

• safety seal • hives • package label • anaphylaxis • by mouth • skin
• antihistamines • consciousness • to treat • itchy eyes • blister package
• hay fever • improve • tongue

Loratadine

Loratadine is used to temporarily relieve the symptoms of .... (allergy to pollen, dust, or other substances in the air) and other allergies. These symptoms include sneezing, runny nose, and ...., nose, or throat. Loratadine is also used to treat itching and redness caused by hives. However, loratadine does not prevent hives or other allergic .... reactions. Loratadine is in a class of medications called .... It works by blocking the action of histamine, a substance in the body that causes allergic symptoms.

Loratadine comes as a syrup (liquid), a tablet, and a rapidly disintegrating (dissolving) tablet to take .... It is usually taken once a day with or without food. Follow the directions on the package label carefully, and ask your doctor or pharmacist to explain any part you do not understand. Take loratadine exactly as directed. Do not take more or less of it or take it more often than directed on the .... or recommended by your doctor. If you take more loratadine than directed, you may experience drowsiness.

If you are taking the rapidly disintegrating tablet, follow the package directions to remove the tablet from the .... without breaking the tablet. Do not try to push the tablet through the foil. After you remove the tablet from the blister package, immediately place it on your .... and close your mouth. The tablet will quickly dissolve and can be swallowed with or without water.

Do not use loratadine .... hives that are bruised or blistered, that are an unusual color, or that do not itch. Call your doctor if you have this type of hives.

Stop taking loratadine and call your doctor if your hives do not .... during the first 3 days of your treatment or if your hives last longer than 6 weeks. If you do not know the cause of your hives, call your doctor.

If you are taking loratadine to treat ...., and you develop any of the following symptoms, get emergency medical help right away: difficulty swallowing, speaking, or breathing; swelling in and around the mouth or swelling of the tongue; wheezing; drooling; dizziness; or loss of .... These may be symptoms of a life-threatening allergic reaction called .... If your doctor suspects that you may experience anaphylaxis with your hives, he may prescribe an epinephrine injector (EpiPen). Do not use loratadine in place of the epinephrine injector.

Do not use this medication if the .... is open or torn.

[From www.nlm.nih.gov/medlineplus/druginfo/meds/a697038.html#why]

About WHO

WHO is the directing and coordinating authority for health within the United Nations system. It is responsible for providing leadership on global health matters, shaping the health research agenda, setting norms and standards, articulating evidence-based policy options, providing technical support to countries and monitoring and assessing health trends.

In the 21st century, health is a shared responsibility, involving equitable access to essential care and collective defence against transnational threats.

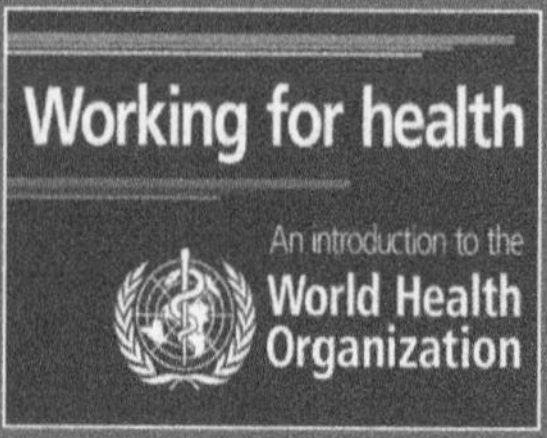

Exercise 7

Give the Italian for:

1. Itching and redness ....
2. By mouth ....
3. The tablet can be swallowed ....
4. Drowsiness ....
5. Life-threatening allergic reaction ....
6. Follow the package directions ....

Pay attention

Advice ➢ consiglio, parere, non significa avviso (uncountable)
Avviso: *warning, announcement* (annuncio), *advertisement* (pubblicità)

Sensitivity, sensitive ➢ sensibile
He is sensitive to my problem/sensitive to cold, pain, light/sensitive microscope/sensitive skin.
or suscettibile
He is sensitive about his origins.

Sensibility, sensible ➢ rilevante
A sensible difference
sensibile, consapevole
Sensible of other people's troubles.

Rational ➢ based on reasons rather than emotions, reasonable

Percepibile ➢ sensible phenomena

Effective ➢ efficace. **Effettivo:** *actual, real.*

UNIT 8

CAREERS IN PHARMACY

BEING A PHARMACIST IN THE UK

A pharmacist is the member of the health team who knows most about all aspects of medicines.

One of the most important advances in health care has been the development of highly specific and effective medicines – medicines that have virtually eliminated some diseases which were major killers in the recent past, and that have reduced the impact of many others.
Pharmacists are the professionists legally responsible for the supply of medicines. Their clinical role is concerned with medicines management, which seeks to improve health through the best use of medicines.
Pharmacists work in:

- community pharmacies;
- GPs surgeries;
- hospitals;
- industry;
- government;
- universities.

How Do You Become a Pharmacist?

To be able to use the title of pharmacist in the UK, you must be registered with the Royal Pharmaceutical Society of Great Britain.
Membership is granted to graduates with a degree in pharmacy from a UK university who have completed a year's training at an approved establishment and passed a registration exam set by the Society.
Training is usually arranged as either 12 months in a hospital or community pharmacy, but it can be done for 6 months in the pharmaceutical industry and 6 months in either hospital or community pharmacy.
Pharmacy offers a variety of interesting careers. Pharmacists can work in a range of positions, with the possibility of flexible working across several of the sectors. Students taking a degree in pharmacy can feel confident that they are starting on a career in which there will always be a need for their services.

Community Pharmacy

Three out of five pharmacists practise in community pharmacy. They will either own a pharmacy ("chemist's shop") or be employed to manage and provide professional services within one.

The duties of a community pharmacist involve supplying medicine for prescriptions, managing medicine for minor ailments of members of the public and giving advice on medicines. They also provide screening services and extra services to patients who are housebound.
Many community pharmacists also provide a pharmaceutical service to nursing and care homes, involving medication reviews and advice on storage and administration of medicines. Some also work with general practitioners (GPs) on a sessional basis, for example, to develop more cost-effective prescribing and practice formularies.

Hospital Pharmacy

Hospital pharmacists work on hospital wards or in outpatient clinics. Most hospital pharmacists specialise in a clinical area, such as paediatrics or intensive care, where they can work towards consultant status.
Working as a hospital pharmacist, practitioners spend a lot of their time on wards with patients and other healthcare professionals as they work with doctors and nurses as part of a multidisciplinary patient-care team.

Primary Care

Primary-care pharmacists work in GP practices. They do not provide a dispensing service, but work with GPs in developing practice formularies and more cost-effective and patient-centred prescribing.
They are involved in a range of services, including drug use reviews, running clinics such as those for cholesterol monitoring, and reviewing the medication of patients on complex drug regimens. They normally have access to patients' notes and medication profile.

Pharmaceutical Advisors

Pharmaceutical advisors' duties include analysing prescribing data at Primary care Trust (PCT) and GP-level, and development of prescribing policy and guidance to GPs on improving the cost-effectiveness of their prescribing.
Many pharmaceutical advisors also advise PCTs on the development of community pharmacy services and on commissioning secondary care services where drug treatments are pivotal.

Pharmaceutical Industry

As well as developing new drugs, the pharmaceutical industry is responsible for the production of existing drugs, ensuring that they are safe, effective and of the highest quality.
Pharmacists are found in all areas of the industry. They use specialist knowledge and skills while keeping a broad view of drug treatment.
The range of roles for pharmacists includes:
- research;
- medical information;
- pharmacovigilance (monitoring product safety);
- regulatory affairs (obtaining product licenses from health authorities);
- medical writing;
- manufacturing and quality control;

- clinical trial supplies;
- sales;
- national and international marketing;
- general management.

Industrial pharmacists have considerable interaction with colleagues, academic researchers, clinicians and other NHS personnel.

Other Careers

Pharmacists can also work in:

- medical journalism;
- forensic service;
- the armed forces;
- VSO (voluntary service overseas);
- universities;
- the NHS;
- National Institute of Clinical Excellence (NICE);
- agricultural and veterinary pharmacy.

[*The University of Manchester*, web site www.pharmacy.manchester.ac.uk]

WORD FILE

- **Care home:** a building where people who are old or ill live.
- **Clinic:** a place, often in a hospital, where medical treatment is given to people who do not need to stay in the hospital.(US): a place where medical treatment is given at a low cost. A group of doctors who work together and share the same offices.
- **Formulary:** collection of formulas for making medicinal preparations.
- **General Practitioner (GP):** a general practitioner or GP is a medical practitioner who provides primary care and specializes in family medicine (UK).
- **Housebound:** not able to leave his own house, especially because he is ill or old.
- **Outpatient:** someone who goes to a hospital for treatment but does not stay for the night: *Outpatient clinic.*
- **Physician:** a healthcare professional licensed to practice medicine. A licensed medical practitioner (US).
- **Practice:** the work of a doctor or lawyer or the place where they work (*Joe had a legal practice in New York*).
- **Practise (to):** to work in a job or profession, especially law or medicine. *To practice* (American English).
- **Primary care:** basic medical treatment that you receive from a doctor who is not a specialist (*Primary care physician*).
- **Ward:** a large room, or a number of rooms, in a hospital where people who need medical tratment stay: maternity, general, geriatric etc., ward.

- **Forensic medicine:** medicina legale.
- **Forensic science:** scienza forense.
- **Pivotal:** cruciale.
- **Storage:** accantonamento, immagazzinamento.
- **Three out of five:** 3 su 5.
- **Ailment:** disturbo, indisposizione.

Exercise 1

Decide which statements are true (T) or false (F).

		T	F
1.	Some diseases have been eliminated thanks to effective medicines.		
2.	Pharmacists can work in the armed forces.		
3.	You need to have a degree in pharmacy to be registered in the Royal Pharmaceutical Society of Great Britain.		
4.	The training for pharmacists can be either 12 months or 6.		
5.	Three out of five pharmacists practise in Hospital pharmacy.		
6.	Pharmaceutical advisors work with GPs in developing practice formularies.		

Exercise 2

Translate the fragments in italics into English.

1. They are *coinvolti in una serie di servizi*, includine drug use reviews, running *ambulatori come quelli per il monitoraggio del colesterolo.*

   ....

   ....

   ....

2. *I doveri degli informatori farmaceutici* include analysing prescribing data at Primary Care Trust.

   ....

   ....

   ....

3. Hospital pharmacists work on *reparti ospedalieri o in ambulatori in day hospital.*

   ....

   ....

   ....

4. *L'iscrizione (all'associazione) è garantita ai laureati* in pharmacy from a UK university who have completed *un tirocinio di un anno* at an approved establishment and *superato* a registration exam.

   ....

   ....

   ....

5. Pharmacists are the professionals legally responsible *per la fornitura di medicine.* Their clinical role is concerned *con la gestione delle medicine, che cerca di migliorare* health through the best use of medicines.

   ....

   ....

   ....

BEING A PHARMACIST IN THE USA

Occupational Outlook Handbook

Nature of the Work

Pharmacists distribute prescription drugs to individuals. They also advise their patients, as well as physicians and other health practitioners, on the selection, dosages, interactions, and side effects of medications. Pharmacists monitor the health and progress of patients to ensure the safe and effective use of medication. Compounding – the actual mixing of ingredients to form medications – is a small part of a pharmacist's practice, because most medicines are produced by pharmaceutical companies in a standard dosage and drug delivery form. Most pharmacists work in a community setting, such as a retail drugstore, or in a health care facility, such as hospital, nursing home, mental health institution, or neighborhood health clinic.

Pharmacists in community pharmacies dispense medications, counsel patients on the use of prescription and over-the-counter medications, and advise physicians about patients' medication therapy. They also advise patients about general health topics such as diet, exercise, and stress management, and provide information on products such as durable medical equipment or home health care supplies. In addition, they may complete third-party insurance forms and other paperwork. Those who own or manage community pharmacies may sell non-health-related merchandise, hire and supervise personnel, and oversee the general operation of the pharmacy. Some community pharmacists provide specialized services to help patients with conditions such as diabetes, asthma, smoking cessation, or high blood pressure; others are also trained to administer vaccinations.

Pharmacists in health care facilities dispense medications and advise the medical staff on the selection and effects of drugs. They may make sterile solutions to be administered intravenously. They also plan, monitor and evaluate drug programs or regimens. They may counsel hospitalized patients on the use of drugs before the patients are discharged.

Increasingly, pharmacists are pursuing nontraditional pharmacy work. Some are involved in research for pharmaceutical manufacturers, developing new drugs and testing their effects. Others work in marketing or sales, providing clients with expertise on the use, effectiveness, and possible side effects of drugs. Some pharmacists work for health insurance companies, developing pharmacy benefit packages and carrying out cost-benefit analyses on certain drugs. Other pharmacists work for the government, managed care organizations, public health care services, the armed services, or pharmacy associations. Finally, some pharmacists are employed full time or part time as college faculty, teaching classes and performing research in a wide range of areas.

Exercise 3

Complete the sentences according to the text.

1. They also .... their patients, as well as .... and other health practitioners, on the selection, ..., interactions, and side effects of medications.
2. Compounding – the actual mixing of .... to form medications – is a small part of a pharmacist's ...., because most medicines are produced by pharmaceutical companies in a standard dosage and drug ....

3. Most pharmacists work in a community ...., such as a retail drugstore, or in a health care ...., such as hospital, ... home, mental health institution, or neighborhood health clinic.
4. Increasingly, pharmacists are .... nontraditional pharmacy work. Some are involved in research for pharmaceutical ...., developing new drugs and testing their effects. Others work in marketing or sales, providing clients with .... on the use, ..., and possible side effects of drugs.
5. Pharmacists in .... care facilities dispense medications and advise the medical .... on the selection and effects of drugs. They may make sterile solutions to be .... intravenously. They also plan, ... and .... drug programs or regimens

Education and Training

Pharmacists must earn a Pharm.D. degree from an accredited college or school of pharmacy. The Pharm.D. degree has replaced the Bachelor of Pharmacy degree, which is no longer being awarded. To be admitted to a Pharm.D. program, an applicant must have completed at least 2 years of postsecondary study, although most applicants have completed 3 or more years. Other entry requirements usually include courses in mathematics and natural sciences, such as chemistry, biology, and physics, as well as courses in the humanities and social sciences.

About 70 percent of Pharm.D. programs require applicants to take the Pharmacy College Admissions Test (PCAT).

Courses offered at colleges of pharmacy are designed to teach students about all aspects of drug therapy. In addition, students learn how to communicate with patients and other health care providers about drug information and patient care. Students also learn professional ethics, concepts of public health, and medication distribution systems management. In addition to receiving classroom instruction, students in Pharm.D. programs spend about one-forth of their time in a variety of pharmacy practice settings under the supervision of licensed pharmacists.

WORD FILE

- **Alumnus:** (pl. alumni) a former student of a school, college, university.
- **Education:** the process by which a person's mind and character are developed through teaching, or through formal instruction at a school or college.
- **Fellowship:** (UK) (countable) a job at a university which involves making a detailed study of a particular subject especially American English money given to some students to allow them to continue their studies at an advanced level (scholarship) (*Giovanni came to the United States on a Fulbright fellowship*).
- **Graduate:** someone who has completed a university degree, especially a first degree. *Undergraduate:* a college student who has not yet earned a degree (*A Harvard graduate, a graduate of Edinburgh University, university graduates, a history graduate*). *To graduate in* (*He's a graduate in philosophy*). *A high-school graduate:* American English someone who has completed the high school.
- **Polite:** having good manners, correct social behaviour. *Politeness.* Opposite: rude.

- **To pursue an education:** perseguire un progetto in campo formativo (istruzione).

The master-of-science degree or the Ph.D. degree are awarded after the completion of a Pharm.D. degree and are designed for those who want additional clinical, laboratory, and research experience. Areas of graduate study include pharmaceutics and pharmaceutical chemistry (physical and chemical properties of drugs and dosage forms), pharmacology (effects of drugs on the body), and pharmacy administration. Many master's and Ph.D. degree holders go on to do research for a drug company or teach at a university.

Other options for pharmacy graduates who are interested in further training include 1-year or 2-year residency programs or fellowships. Pharmacy residencies are postgraduate training programs in pharmacy practice and usually require the completion of a research project. These programs are often mandatory for pharmacists who wish to work in hospitals. Pharmacy fellowships are highly individualized programs that are designed to prepare participants to work in a specialized area of pharmacy.

A pharmacist is someone whose job is to prepare and sells medicines in a shop or hospital. This is the usual word in (US), but in (UK) pharmacist is slightly technical and it is more usual to use the word chemist. The place where a pharmacist works is a pharmacy. This can be a shop, part of a shop, or part of a hospital. Pharmacy is the usual word in (US). In (UK), you usually refer to the part of a hospital that prepares and gives out medicines as a pharmacy, but the usual word for a shop where medicines are prepared and sold is a chemist or a chemist's. In Britain chemists usually sell also other things, such as beauty or baby products. A shop like this in the US is called a drugstore.

Licensure

A license to practice pharmacy is required in all States, the District of Columbia, and all US territories. To obtain a license, a prospective pharmacist must graduate from a college of pharmacy that is accredited by the ACPE and pass a series of examinations. All States, US territories, and the District of Columbia require the North American Pharmacist Licensure Exam (NAPLEX), which tests pharmacy skills and knowledge.

Exercise 4

Decide which statements are true (T) or false (F).

		T	F
1.	Pharmacists can obtain a license after a university degree.	☐	☐
2.	The Bachelor of Pharmacy Degree is not in use any longer.	☐	☐
3.	Applicants to a Pharm. D. program are supposed to have completed 2 years of post secondary school.	☐	☐
4.	One-fourth of a Pharm. D. program is spent in learning professional ethics.	☐	☐
5.	A license can be required in many States.	☐	☐

Exercise 5

Read carefully and fill in the blanks with the future tense of the suggested verbs. (Pay attention! Verbs are used more times and can be in a passive form too.)

• to continue • to grow • to need • to lead • to increase • to offer

Job outlook

Employment change. Employment of pharmacists is expected to grow by 17 percent between 2008 and 2018, which is faster than the average for all occupations. The increasing numbers of middle-aged and elderly people – who use more prescription drugs than younger people – .... to spur demand for pharmacists throughout the projection period. In addition, as scientific advances lead to new drug products, and as an increasing number of people obtain prescription drug coverage, the need for these workers .... to expand.

Pharmacists also are becoming more involved in patient care. As prescription drugs become more complex, and as the number of people taking multiple medications increases, the potential for dangerous drug interactions .... Pharmacists .... to counsel patients on the proper use of medication, assist in drug selection and dosage, and monitor complex drug regimens. This need .... to rapid growth for pharmacists in medical care establishments, such as doctors' offices, outpatient care centers, and nursing care facilities.

Demand also .... in mail-order pharmacies, which often are more efficient than pharmacies in other practice settings. Employment also .... to grow in hospitals, drugstores, grocery stores, and mass retailers, because pharmacies in these settings .... to process the majority of all prescriptions and increasingly .... patient care services, such as the administration of vaccines.

Pay attention

A large number of people obtains. *A large number of people obtain.*

In American English si preferisce concordare il verbo con il sostantivo plurale invece che con quello singolare di tipo collettivo.

HOSPITAL PHARMACY

The professionals concerned with health care work together as a team. Nowhere is this more evident than in the hospital services. A person taking up the career of hospital pharmacist can be assured of a challenging and interesting job, one that changes rapidly in response to developments in the health care field. The pharmacist must be able to integrate well with co-workers, for example, doctors, nurses, radiologists etc.

The pharmacist is primarily responsible for supplying medicines as efficiently and economically as possible; for their secure and proper storage and for their distribution throughout the hospital. The quality, safety and use of medicines must be closely monitored by the pharmacist. This usually entails involvement at ward level. It requires constant updating to keep abreast with the many new or reformulated products being developed by medical and pharmaceutical researchers.

The hospital pharmacy is the centre of drug information. The pharmacist is expected to lecture nurses and medical students on the action of drugs, dose rates, side effects and related problems. They act on the drug therapeutic committees where overall policy is determined in relation to drug usage, new products, clinical trials, infection control, the hospital formulary etc. The pharmacist increasingly plays a vital role in clinical budgeting and on finance committees.

While most medicines nowadays are formulated and prepackaged by the pharmaceutical industry, medications may have to be individually prepared for particular patients. The pharmacist must retain the traditional compounding skills to meet these requirements. Even with modern innova-

tions, there is still a significant demand for this service. It is also important in the preparation of sterile products and of disinfectants.
The career structure in hospital pharmacy provides for an increasing degree of responsibility. The pharmacist, after a year's post-graduate experience, enters the service at the basic grade. With time, he or she moves from basic to senior grade and then either to Chief II or Chief I status. In normal circumstances, promotion can be achieved in a reasonable time scale.

Exercise 6

Read the text and answer the questions.

1. What is a hospital pharmacist responsible for?

....

....

....

2. Why is he requested to be constantly up-dated?

....

....

....

3. What is a hospital pharmacist expected to do as far as information is concerned?

....

....

....

4. Give a short description of a hospital pharmacist's duties.

....

....

....

Exercise 7

Give the Italian for.

1. Health care field. ....
2. Secure and proper storage. ....
3. Most medicines are formulated and prepackaged. ....
4. An increasing degree of responsibility. ....
5. Involvement at ward level. ....

Exercise 8

Complete according to the text.

1. An increasingly vital role is ....
2. The monitoring of .... is provided ....
3. Working as a team is particularly ....
4. Medications for particular patients ....

PHARMACEUTICAL SALES REPRESENTATIVE

Job Overview

Pharmaceutical representatives, also known as drug reps or pharmaceutical salespeople, provide drug information and product samples to physicians. Also, pharmaceutical reps monitor prescribing patterns of physicians in a given geographic territory.

As a pharmaceutical representative, one would typically represent a particular drug or group of drugs, and would meet with physicians who specialize in the applicable medical field. For example, a drug rep who manages a territory for a drug which treats heartburn would most likely call on gastroenterologists and internists.

Typical Work Week and Environment for Pharmaceutical Sales Reps

A drug rep may work out of a home based office and a company car. They may be required to check in at a regional or local office. However, most of the rep's time will be spent in their territory, or "in the field" meeting with physicians, or attempting to meet with them by visiting the physicians' practices. Therefore, a potential rep should be very comfortable being in a car much of the day, traveling to anywhere from four to eight physicians' offices daily.

In addition to the daily physician visits, reps may be required to attend sales meetings, conference calls, or training sessions with the management team. Drug reps may also do lunchtime presentations at physicians' offices, supplying lunch for the office staff and discussing the drug's indications, side effects, features, and benefits.

Education Requirements

Most pharmaceutical companies prefer to hire college graduates with at least a bachelor's degree, and many of the big companies look for the top graduates and top performers of the class.

Skill Requirements

In addition to the college degree, pharmaceutical reps must be very polished, professional, and well-spoken. They must be highly organized in order to manage their territory and time optimally. Additionally, reps must have the ability to memorize vast amounts of medical terminology and detailed information about the medication they represent, and be able to intelligently relay the information to physicians. Pharma sales can be stressful, so they must be able to handle the pressure of meeting productivity goals and deadlines.

What's to Like

There are many reasons why pharmaceutical jobs are coveted by many aspiring job seekers in the medical industry. The earning potential for pharmaceutical reps is strong, especially when compared to other sales jobs. Also the perks are good such as the company car, trips, bonuses, and benefits such as medical, tuition reimbursement, retirement, 401k, etc. Additionally, if you establish yourself as a successful rep, your career track options will multiply and you can have a very long, successful, lucrative career.

What's Not to Like about Pharmaceutical Sales Jobs

The days of the cushy pharmaceutical sales jobs are over. Due to the abundance of companies, drugs, and reps in the industry, and also due to the continual push for doctors to see more patients in less time, many physicians refuse to speak with reps on a regular basis. Other physicians have significantly cut back on the time they will spend with drug reps and which ones they will meet. Pharma reps must be patient and persistent when working in their territories to speak with as many physicians as possible. Often, reps may spend more time in the waiting room than in front of a physician.

In the past, pharmaceutical reps frequently enjoyed entertaining doctors at high-end dinners, concerts, and resorts. Although the perks are still great for pharma reps, there has been somewhat of a "crackdown" on the sales tactics of big pharmaceutical companies. Therefore, the activities of the reps are tracked much more carefully than they were in past years. Additionally, modern technology such as electronic signature pads and GPS tracking on the company cars has caused reps to be held much more accountable for their whereabouts on an hourly and daily basis.

Career Path and Advancement for Pharmaceutical Sales Reps

Pharmaceutical representatives who wish to advance into management roles have a variety of choices. There are many levels of management and a variety of departments within most established pharmaceutical companies. For example, a sales rep can become a district or regional manager, or a Director of Sales, then Senior Director, on up to Vice President. Additionally, reps can transition among various departments and manage different drugs and drug launches. Once you work your way up the chain, you may have to consider relocation to the headquarters, so be prepared to hit a ceiling or move. There are drug companies headquartered in a variety of locations nationwide, but California and New Jersey are major hubs, along with the midwestern region of the US.

WORD FILE

- **Hub:** a central node in a network. The term comes from the analogy to a wheel's hub, the center.
- **Perk:** an incidental benefit awarded for certain types of employment (*car, pc etc.*) also called *fringe benefits.*

- **Covet (to):** ambire, desiderare.
- **Headquarters:** sede centrale.
- **Whereabouts:** percorsi.

Exercise 9

Fill in the gaps with a suitable word from the passage.

In addition to the college ...., pharmaceutical reps must be very polished, professional, and well-spoken. They must be highly .... in order to manage their territory and time optimally. Additionally, reps must have the ability to memorize vast amounts of medical .... and detailed information about the medication they represent, and be able to intelligently relay the information to .... Pharma sales can be stressful, so they must be able to handle the pressure of meeting productivity .... and deadlines.

There are many reasons why pharmaceutical jobs are coveted by many aspiring job .... in the medical industry. The earning potential for pharmaceutical reps is strong, especially when compared to other .... jobs. Also the .... are good such as the company car, trips, bonuses, and benefits such as medical, tuition reimbursement, retirement, 401k, etc.

Exercise 10

Give a job description of a Pharmaceutical Sales Reps (in about 60 words).

....

....

....

....

....

....

....

....

....

....

....

Exercise 11

Give a list of the required skills.

....

....

....

....

....

....

....

....

....

....

Exercise 12

Answer the following questions.

1. What is the attitude of physicians towards reps?

   ....

   ....

   ....

   ....

2. Which are the possibilities of advancement for a pharmaceutical rep?

   ....

   ....

   ....

   ....

UNIT 9

JOBS AND POSITIONS

APPLYING FOR A JOB

After you have found some jobs that interest you, the next step is to apply for them. Many potential employers require complete resumes or application forms and cover letters. Later, you will probably need to go on interviews to meet with employers face to face.

Resumes and Application Forms

Resumes and application forms give employers written evidence of your qualifications and skills. The goal of these documents is to prove – as clearly and directly as possible – how your qualifications match the job's requirements. Do this by highlighting the experience, accomplishments, education, and skills that most closely fit the job you want.

Gathering information. Resumes and application forms both include the same information. As a first step, gather the following facts:

- *Contact information*, including your name, mailing address, e-mail address (if you have one you check often), and telephone number;
- *Type of work* or specific job you are seeking or a qualifications summary, which describes your best skills and experience in just a few lines;
- *Education*, including school name and its city and State, months and years of attendance, highest grade completed or diploma or degree awarded, and major subject or subjects studied. Also consider listing courses and awards that might be relevant to the position;
- *Experience*, paid and volunteer. For each job, include the job title, name and location of employer, and dates of employment. Briefly describe your job duties and major accomplishments. In a resume, use phrases instead of sentences to describe your work; write, for example, "Supervised 10 children" instead of writing "I supervised 10 children";
- *Special skills*. You might list computer skills, proficiency in foreign languages, achievements, or membership in organizations in a separate section;
- *References*. Be ready to provide references if requested. Good references could be former employers, coworkers, or teachers or anyone else who can describe your abilities and job-related traits. You will be asked to provide contact information for the people you choose.

Throughout the application or resume, focus on accomplishments that relate most closely to the job you want. You can even use the job announcement as a guide, using some of the same words and phrases to describe your work and education.

Look for concrete examples that show your skills. When describing your work experience, for instance, you might say that you increased sales by 10 percent, finished a task in half the usual time, or received three letters of appreciation from customers.

Choosing a Format

After gathering the information you want to present, the next step is to put it in the proper format. In an application form, the format is set. Just fill in the blanks. But make sure you fill it out completely and follow all instructions. Do not omit any requested information. Consider making a copy of the form before filling it out, in case you make a mistake and have to start over. If possible, have someone else look over the form before submitting it.

In a resume, there are several acceptable ways of organizing the information you want to include. It is common to place the most important information first. One format is to list the applicant's past jobs in reverse chronological order, describing the most recent employment first and working backward. But some applicants use a functional format, organizing their work experience under headings that describe their major skills. They then include a brief work history section that lists only job titles, employers, and dates of employment. Still other applicants choose a format that combines these two approaches in some way. Choose the style that best showcases your skills and experience. Examples of resume formats can be found on the Web sites of career centers, job boards, and State employment services.

Whatever format you choose, keep your resume short. Many experts recommend that new workers use a one-page resume. Avoid long blocks of text and italicized material. Consider using bullets to highlight duties or key accomplishments.

Before submitting your resume, make sure that it is easy to read. Are the headings clear and consistently formatted with bold or some other style of type? Is the type face large enough? Much like application forms, it is useful to ask someone to proofread your resume for spelling and other errors. In addition, use your computer's spell checker.

Keep in mind that some employers scan resumes into databases, which they then search for specific keywords or phrases. The keywords are usually nouns referring to experience, education, personal characteristics, or industry buzz words. Identify keywords by reading the job description and qualifications in the job ad; use these same words in your resume. For example, if the job description includes customer service tasks, use the words "customer service" on your resume. Scanners sometimes misread paper resumes, which could mean some of your keywords don't get into the database. So, if you know that your resume will be scanned, and you have the option, e-mail an electronic version. If you must submit a paper resume, make it scannable by using a simple font and avoiding underlines, italics, and graphics.

Cover Letters

When sending a resume, most people include a cover letter to introduce themselves to the prospective employer. Most cover letters are no more than three short paragraphs. Your cover letter should capture the employer's attention, follow a business letter format, and usually should include the following information:

- name and address of the specific person to whom the letter is addressed;
- reason for your interest in the company or position;
- your main qualifications for the position;
- request for an interview;
- your home and work telephone numbers.

If you send a scannable resume, you should also include a scannable cover letter, which avoids graphics, fancy fonts, italics, and underlines.

[From www.bls.gov/oco/ocos325.htm]

Exercise 1

Complete according to the text.

1. A resumé must contain details about:

- ....
- ....
- ....
- ....
- ....
- ....

2. One format is to list ....
3. Keep your resumé ....
4. Avoid ....
5. Consider using ....
6. The keywords are ....
7. A cover letter should include the following information:

- ....
- ....
- ....
- ....
- ....
- ....

WORD FILE

- **Employ (to):** to pay someone to work for you.
- **Employee:** someone that is paid to work for someone else (*A government employee*).
- **Employment:** the condition of having a paid job.
- **Employer:** a person, company or organization that employs people.
- **Proofread (to):** to read through something in order to correct any mistakes in it.

- **Accomplishment:** realizzazione, compimento.
- **Award:** riconoscimento, premio.
- **Bold:** neretto, grassetto ma anche audace, sfacciato.
- **Bullet:** proiettile (qui sta per bullet point: indicatore grafico).
- **Buzz words:** espressioni attuali, di moda.
- **Coworker:** compagno di lavoro, collega.
- **Former:** precedente.
- **Line:** riga, fila, linea.
- **Misread (to):** interpretare erroneamente.
- **Phrase:** espressione.
- **Proper:** appropriato. Proprio: own.
- **Reverse:** inverso.
- **Sentence:** frase.

A curriculum vitae (CV) is an account of a person's education, qualifications and working experiences.
It should be written in a simple and concise form with clearly separate items:
It is supposed to be typed and sent with a covering letter which may be asked to be hand written.
It is called "résumé" in the USA.
The layout may vary according to the country or the specific requirements of a company or institution.
In the USA, for example, it does not usually include information about one's marital status.
Tips for a curriculum:
- keep it simple;
- lay it out chronologically;
- write dates in full.

CURRICULUM VITAE

Name:	Charles W. Tiberlake
Born:	Dundee – 29 September 1982
Address:	34, Melville Rd. Cambridge N2 4W
Mail address:	cw.tib@yahoo.uk
Marital Status:	single
Education:	Graduate in Pharmacy at the Leichester University. A one year course in "Pharmaceutical care economics" at the Georgetown University. A three months course in "Evaluating new drugs" at the Sullivan Centre of Reading.
Foreign Languages:	English mother tongue. Fluent in Spanish.

DR. PERHAN'S STORY

Dr. Perhan was born in New York City on nov. 2, 1954. Married with 3 children he lives now in Boston, Ma.
Graduated at the New York University School of Medicine he received his master and PhD at the University of Washington.
Dr. Perhan is the Simon Gelman Professor of Anaesthesia (Biochemistry and Molecular Pharmacology) at Harvard Medical School, and is Professor in the Department of Oral Medicine, Infection and Immunity at Harvard School of Dental Medicine and an Affiliate Faculty Member of MIT. Dr. Perhan received post-doctoral training in Physiological Chemistry at the Karolinska Institute Medical University (Stockholm, Sweden) with Prof. Bengt Samuelsson (1982 Nobel Laureate in Medicine). He was appointed to the Harvard Faculty in 1986 and has served as Senior Biochemist in Medicine at Brigham and Women's Hospital since 1992.
He has received a number of awards and honors. In July 2000, he received a MERIT Award from the National Institute of General Medical Sciences; an honorary degree in 1996 from Harvard University. In April 2000, he received the distinction of being named the first "Endowed Distinguished Scientist" at BWH. Dr. Perhan received the MacArthur Research Service Award in 2003. He was the 2005 Kreshover Lecturer at NIH (NIDCR) and received the LSU Chancellor's Award in Neuroscience in 2006. Dr. Perhan has authored 206 publications.

Dr. Perhan research studies focus on structural elucidation of bioactive molecules of interest in acute inflammation. The overall mission is "To identify novel mediators, pathways, and cellular targets critical in regulating and promoting resolution of inflammation and their relation to human disease." Recently these studies focused on structural elucidation of novel molecules and pathways that serve as pro-resolving and/or endogenous anti-inflammatory chemical signals.

Dr. Perhan elucidated several new families of lipid-derived, local-acting chemical mediators, coined the Resolvins and Protectins, as well as their endogenous aspirin-triggered forms that dampen inflammatory responses. He has also designed novel therapeutic approaches using some of these structures as biotemplates. New therapeutic approaches built with the knowledge of these biochemical signaling pathways could be more potent and better tolerated since they are based on structures of endogenous natural compounds. Also, since the central nervous system is rich in DHA, the novel neuroprotectins may have a physiological role in protecting neural tissues from inflammation-initiated injury.

When he is not conducting research or teaching Dr Perhan enjoys spending time with his family sharing with them his love for travelling to new places.

Reading historical novels is one of his favorite hobbies. Skiing is his favorite sport and Colorodo provides him with beautiful slopes.

Exercise 2

Read about Dr. Perhan and then fill in the CV form.

First name: ....

Surname: ....

Place of birth: ....

Place of residence: ....

Marital status: ....

Present position: ....

....

Education: ....

....

Academic titles: ....

....

Awards: ....

....

Research achievements: ....

....

....

Present field of research: ....

....

....

Favorite spare time occupations: ....

....

WORD FILE

- **Salary:** money that an employee receives for the work he/she does. It is usually paid every month.
- **Wages:** money earned by workers usually in non-professional jobs.

- **Amazing:** sorprendente, meraviglioso. *To amaze:* sorprendere, stupire.
- **Appoint (to):** nominare, assegnare.
- **Dampen (to):** soffocare, smorzare.
- **Grow up (to):** crescere, diventare adulti. *To grow:* aumentare, crescere, coltivare.
- **Injury:** ferita, lesione.
- **Involvement:** coinvolgimento. *To involve:* coinvolgere.
- **Position:** posto di lavoro.
- **Raise (to):** alzare, sollevare, allevare.
- **Recruitment:** assunzione, ricerca di personale.
- **Seeking for a job:** cercare lavoro.
- **To pursue an education:** perseguire un progetto in campo formativo (istruzione).

ELEMENTS OF A LETTER

Letterhead

Generally positioned on the left top side. It's the address of the writer. (Found on the right side too.)

Date

Don't mention the town before the date. Don't write the months in figures:
16th May, 2007/16 May 2007/May 16, 2007.

Address

Generally on the right side: *Mr Steve Wright*, *Mrs Jennifer Jones*, *Miss Kate Wilson*, *Ms Susan Baker* generally used instead of Mrs or Miss. Messers (Messieurs): used before all firms trading under a person's proper name *Messers Richard Blank & sons*. *The*-institutions, names containing words such as company, centre, university, department etc.: *The Chemical Institute of Maryland, The Pharmacy Department of.*

Salutation

To the reader of the letter:
Dear Mr Fox/Dear Ms Turner, *Dear Sir/Madam* when you do not know the name.
Sir/Madam: very formal.
Dear Sir (USA): letters addressed to companies or institutions.

Complimentary close

Yours faithfully
Yours sincerely
Best regards (less formal)
Yours truly (USA)
Truly yours (USA), *Sincerely yours* (USA)
Sincerely (USA).

Signature

It's placed under the complimentary close. The position of the writer or its typed name is placed under the signature.

10 Bath Place,
Winchester,
S022 5HH
January 23, 2...

The Pharmfinders Ltd,
Suite 109/110, Lovell House,
Birchwood Park,
Warrington,WA3 6FW.
UK

With reference to your advertisement on your website (ref.) I wish to apply for the position of Pharmacy Manager.

As you can see from the enclosed Curriculum Vitae, I graduated from Manchester University in Pharmacy and I attended a one year course in Pharmacological Chemistry at the University of Bath.

For the past four years I have been working in three different health center pharmacies belonging to the same multiple group. In my present post I have acquired considerable experience and I have learnt how to run a pharmacy.

The reason why I am looking for another job is my desire to improve my situation by working for a bigger company with better prospects.

I hope you will take my application into consideration.

Yours sincerely,

Kathryn Ann Lee
Encl.

Exercise 3

This is the presentation of the Pharmfinders Ltd. Read it and answer the questions.

Pharmfinders are the UK's leading pharmacist recruitment agency
We provide expert career advice and access to a wide variety of UK pharmacy vacancies. We manage hundreds of pharmacist jobs for a variety of different community, industry and private hospital employers. Our team of experienced **pharmacist recruitment** consultants will assist you throughout the entire recruitment process ensuring your options are fully considered and your chances of success optimised.
Pharmfinders help more pharmacists get employed pharmacist jobs in the UK than any other recruitment agency. Our entirely FREE, no obligation, career guidance service is available to any UK registered or eligible pharmacist interested in understanding more about the UK **pharmacist jobs** market.

Pharmacy jobs are plentiful in many areas of the UK but identifying those **pharmacy vacancies** and companies suited to your particular skills, circumstances and aspirations is what we are all about. As a pharmacist recruitment agency we work with some of the UK's leading FTSE 100 companies and private medical providers as well as smaller independently owned and start up businesses. The common link is that they all have **pharmacist jobs in the UK**. So if it's anything to do with **pharmacy jobs**, Pharmfinders should be your first port of call.

Tick [ ] in which cases you should address to the Pharmfinders?

To find a job as a pharmacist. [ ]
To find pharmacies on sale in the Uk. [ ]
To recruit pharmacists for oversea jobs. [ ]
To require the search of a pharmacist suitable for the necessities of your company or firm. [ ]

Job detail for: Pharmacy Manager

Job Ref: Pharmacist – North Humberside – 44

Location: Hull, North Humberside

Salary: £37,000 – £55,000 depending on hours/skills/experience

Job Description

Pharmfinders (www.pharmfinders.co.uk) are currently working with a dynamic multiple where recent acquisitions have significantly increased the opportunities available for pharmacists in the group. This is an exciting time in the company's development as they exploit the opportunities created through their enlarged operations and a significant brand awareness media campaign. We are currently recruiting a Pharmacy Managers for their health centre pharmacy in HULL. On offer is an excellent salary (negotiable depending upon skills and experience) and a first class benefits package including 25 days holiday, bonus, pension, RPSGB fees paid, staff discount and more.

For more information, please contact Pharmfinders on +44 (0) 1625 529 228, or apply by completing our online registration form.

Exercise 4

Decide which statements are true (T) or false (F).

		T	F
1.	The advertisement is about a position in Hull.		
2.	The job is inside a health centre.		
3.	The offered salary is negotiable.		
4.	The benefit package is inclusive of a special discount for the staff.		

WORD FILE

- **Advertisement:** annuncio pubblicitario (ad.). There are two types of press advertisements:
- **Career:** a job or profession for which one is trained and which one intends to follow. General course of a person's work. **Pay attention** non ha alcun significato positivo come in italiano.
- **Charity:** an organization that helps people, money or help given for generosity.
- **Classified ads:** when they appear under a "classified heading" like: jobs, houses, cars etc. and their cost is per line or word.
- **Display ads:** when they cover a full or half page and can contain illustrations.
- **Recruit (to):** to find in order to employ recruitment agency: a business which finds suitable people for employers.
- **Vacancy:** an unfilled place or space. *Vacancies* (of a job): not at present filled.

- **An (on) average:** in media.
- **Applicant:** candidato, richiedente.
- **Awareness:** consapevolezza.
- **Exploit (to):** utilizzare, sfruttare.

Job Ref: Pharmacist - West Sussex - 564
Location: Brighton, West Sussex
Salary: Competitive - depends on hours/skills/experience

Job Description
Pharmfinders (www.pharmfinders.co.uk) are currently looking to recruit a Pharmacist/Pharmacy Manager to work in a private hospital in Brighton. Our client is Britain's largest healthcare charity and has hospitals & wellbeing centres across the UK. With an average of 40 beds, each hospital has modern, comfortable facilities and all the benefits of having a small supportive team. The successful candiate will lead the medicines management and clinical pharmacy aspects of the oncology services. Providing acute care in an independent hospital combines the best of both worlds of patient facing pharmacy and we encourage applicants with either hospital or community background! Training & development will be provided.
For more information, please contact Pharmfinders on +44 (0) 1625 529 228, or apply by completing our online registration form.

Exercise 5

Decide which statements are true (T) or false (F).

	T	F
1. This ad is about a position in a Brighton private hospital.		
2. The hospital owner is a healthcare charity.		
3. The candidate is supposed to be the hospital manager.		
4. The chosen candidate will receive training and development.		

UNIT 10

SCIENTIFIC PAPERS

ABSTRACTS

An abstract is a self-contained, short, and powerful statement that describes a larger work. Components vary according to discipline; an abstract of a social science or scientific work may contain the scope, purpose, results, and contents of the work. An abstract of a humanities work may contain the thesis, background, and conclusion of the larger work. An abstract is not a review, nor does it evaluate the work being abstracted. While it contains key words found in the larger work, the abstract is an original document rather than an extracted passage.

The two most important reasons for writing an abstract are selection and indexing. Abstracts allow readers who may be interested in the longer work to quickly decide whether it is worth their time to read it. Also, many online databases use abstracts to index larger works. Therefore, abstracts should contain keywords and phrases that allow for easy searching

When do people write abstracts?

- when submitting articles to journals, especially online journals;
- when applying for research grants;
- when writing a book proposal;
- when completing the Ph.D. dissertation or MA thesis;
- when writing a proposal for a conference paper;
- when writing a proposal for a book chapter.

There are two types of abstracts: **descriptive** and **informative**.

Descriptive abstracts

A descriptive abstract indicates the type of information found in the work. It makes no judgments about the work, nor does it provide results or conclusions of the research. It does incorporate key words found in the text and may include the purpose, methods, and objectives of the research and it describes the work being abstracted. Descriptive abstracts are usually very short – 250 words or less.

Informative abstracts

A good informative abstract acts as a surrogate for the work itself presenting and explaining all the main arguments and the important results. An informative abstract includes the information that can be found in a descriptive abstract (purpose, methods, scope) but also includes the results and conclusions of the research and the recommendations of the author. An informative abstract is rarely more than 10% of the length of the entire work.

Key Elements for Writing an Abstract

1. **Reason for writing.** What is the importance of the research? Why would a reader be interested in the larger work?
2. **Problem.** What problem does this work attempt to solve? What is the scope of the project? What is the main argument/thesis/claim?
3. **Methodology.** An abstract of a scientific work may include specific models or approaches used in the larger study.
4. **Results.** Again, an abstract of a scientific work may include specific data that indicates the results of the project.
5. **Implications.** What changes should be implemented as a result of the findings of the work? How does this work add to the body of knowledge on the topic?

[this list of elements is adapted with permission from Phil Koopman, "How to Write an Abstract," www.ece.cmu.edu/~koopman/essays/abstract.html]

All abstracts include:

1. The full citation of the source preceding the abstract.
2. The most important information first.
3. The same level of language found in the original, including technical language.
4. Key words and phrases that quickly identify the content and focus of the work.
5. Clear, concise, and powerful language.

Abstracts may include:

1. The thesis of the work in the first sentence.
2. The background that places the work in the larger body of literature.
3. The same chronological structure of the original work.

How not to write an abstract:

1. Do not refer extensively to other works.
2. Do not add information not contained in the original work.
3. Do not define terms.

POSTERS

Introduction

Posters are widely used at a scientific conference as a means of presenting information in a clear and concise way.

Facilities such as word processors, computer graphics packages and desktop publishing have all made the production of posters a much less daunting task.

Posters should:

- be visually attractive
- stimulate interest from their readers
- be displayed in favourable lighting and surroundings
- be legible from distance
- be logically laid out with a format which is easy to follow
- convey their message in a concise way

There is no "standard" structure for a poster. However the best posters, generally follow the guidelines of a published paper with sections like Introduction, Methods, Results and Discussion/ Conclusion/Significance.

3rd INTERNATIONAL SYMPOSIUM
INTEGRATED BIOMARKERS IN CARDIOVASCULAR DISEASE

Seattle, Washington (USA)
Bell Harbor Conference Center

Symposium Description
This symposium is designed to update scientists and clinicians on recent research related to the integration of biomarkers in the clinical treatment of cardiovascular diseases, thereby enhancing patient outcome. In particular, this symposium will provide physicians with a comprehensive update in the field of biomarkers to facilitate the transfer of the use of integrated biomarkers from research centers and clinical centers of excellence to routine application in standard clinical care. The ultimate goal is to improve patient care through the development of well-validated bioimaging and biochemical markers to be used in human pathophysiological conditions and for optimal drug design.

Accreditation
This activity has been planned and implemented in accordance with the Essential Areas and Policies of the Accreditation Council for Continuing Medical Education (ACCME) through the joint sponsorship of the University of Washington School of Medicine and The Giovanni Lorenzini Medical Foundation. The University of Washington School of Medicine is accredited by the ACCME to provide continuing medical education for physicians.
The University of Washington School of Medicine designates this educational activity for a maximum of 18.0 AMA PRA Category 1 Credits™. Physicians should only claim credit commensurate with the extent of their participation in the activity.

Posters
A limited number of posters on topics of specific interest will be accepted by the Scientific Committee. Selected posters will be exhibited for the duration of the symposium. The deadline for the receipt of abstracts is May 15, 2008. The official letter of acceptance, including guidelines for poster presentation will be sent to the presenting author by June 1, 2008. The presenting author must register for the symposium no later than June 15 or the abstract will be omitted from the final program.

Abstract Submission Information
The abstracts should preferably fit into one page, may contain figures, graphs, tables and must be written in English. Abstracts must be submitted in Microsoft Word format, size 12 font and should contain: poster title, name of authors (name of presenter in bold), institution and contact email. Abstracts may be sent as an attachment via email to smm@u.washington.edu or uploaded electronically.

[*Guidelines* prepared by Dr Michael Thomas
Department of Clinical Biochemistry, Royal Free Hospital,
Pond Street, Hampstead, London, adapted from]

WORD FILE

- **Argument:** a reason given to support or disprove something.
- **Humanities:** (the pl.) studies such as ancient and modern literature etc.
- **To be worth:** valere, valer la pena di (*This car is well worth the price. What are fifty dollars worth?*).

Exercise 1

Find out the English corresponding expressions.

1. Quando si fa domanda per sovvenzioni alla ricerca.

   ....

   ....

2. Un'enunciazione che descrive un lavoro più ampio.

   ....

   ....

3. Contiene le parole chiave trovate in un lavoro più ampio.

   ....

   ....

4. Raramente supera il 10% della lunghezza dell'intero lavoro.

   ....

   ....

5. Mezzi quali word processors, pacchetti di computer grafica hanno reso la produzione dei posters un compito molto meno gravoso.

   ....

   ....

6. I posters dovrebbero essere mostrati con una luce favorevole e una favorevole ambientazione.

   ....

   ....

Exercise 2

Answer the following questions.

1. What is an abstract?

   ....

   ....

   ....

2. What is a poster?

   ....

   ....

   ....

Exercise 3

Decide which statements are true (T) or false (F).

	T	F
1. This Symposium is designed to provide scientists and clinicians with the most updated research in the integration of biomarkers in cardiovascular diseases.		
2. Participants will be provided with updated information in the use of biomarkers with the final aim to improve patient care.		
3. The organizing committee would like to receive abstracts which are not more than one page long.		
4. Abstracts are supposed to be sent by mail.		
5. The author and presenter names are requested to be written in bold.		
6. In order to get the abstracts on the final program they are supposed to be sent within June the 15th.		

DRUGGING THE CANCER GENOME

DRUGS AND BIOMARKERS FOR PERSONALISED CANCER MEDICINE

Date: Wednesday 30 May 20.., 2.30pm.

Venue: Whitworth Art Gallery, The University of Manchester, Oxford Road.

Speaker: Professor Paul Workman PhD, FMedSci FIBiol Director of Cancer Research UK for Cancer Therapeutics.

Open to: Staff, researchers and postgraduates of The University of Manchester, Paterson Institute for Cancer Research, and to the staff and invited guests of ICON. Admission is free but subject to registration.

Registration: To register for this event, please email mary.johnson@manchester.ac.uk or telephone +44(0)161 275 2436.

Registration deadline: Thursday 24th May 20..

Abstract

We are currently living through an incredibly exciting and productive era for cancer drug discovery and development. Proof of concept for drugging the cancer genome has been established with approved agents like trastuzumab, imatinib, gefitinib, erlotinib and others. But alongside some spectacular successes and tremendous opportunities there are also enormous challenges.

On the one hand, we have increasing knowledge of the genetic and molecular causation of cancer. On the other hand, the attrition rate for cancer drugs in the clinic remains high, failure often occurs late and survival rates in the major solid tumours have not been extended dramatically.

In this lecture I will aim to capture the sense of excitement and describe the opportunities and challenges in the discovery and design of molecularly targeted small molecule cancer drugs. In particular, I will stress the importance of integrating three key themes:

- targets;
- technologies;
- treatments.

Targets

The molecular targets of contemporary drug discovery projects now reflect our increasing, though still incomplete, understanding of the genes and pathways that are responsible for the initiation and malignant progression of cancer. High-throughput technologies, including gene expression profiling and genome resequencing methods, are accelerating the rate of cancer gene discovery, but also revealing a high level of complexity – for example the occurrence of large numbers of low abundance driver gene mutations across various cancers and the presence of combinations of many mutant genes within individual cancers.
The different ways in which potential new molecular targets can be considered, validated and prioritized will be discussed.

Technologies

The integrated application of a range of powerful drug discovery technologies, including genomics, high-throughput, fragment, computational and other compound screening methodologies, together with chemical and structural biology will be illustrated. Examples of our multidisciplinary small molecule cancer drug discovery will be described (e.g. HSP90, PI3 kinase, AKT/PKB) with emphasis on how the challenges of multi-parameter lead optimization are being met.

Treatments

The new treatments that have been emerging over the last decade are beginning to reflect the success of the new mechanism-based molecular therapeutics that act on cancer-causing targets and that have benefited from technological innovations in drug design. As a result, cancer drugs are leading the way in the development of personalised molecular medicines.
I will illustrate how the development and use of such treatments depends of the identification of biomarkers to select appropriate patients, to monitor the effects of treatment and to develop the best schedule of administration. Decisions can be made based on the organization of biomarkers into a 'pharmacological audit trail.' Future challenges for drugging the cancer genome will be highlighted, including drug resistance, drug combinations, cost and accessibility. Comments will be made on the changing roles of academia, biotech and big pharma. Exciting times.

Professor Paul Workman

[This lecture series, formerly named the Medeval Distinguished Lecture Series, is sponsored by Icon]

WORD FILE

- **Audit:** a detailed examination of something in order to check if it is good enough. *Audit trail:* records which show a series of steps leading to a certain situation.
- **Genome:** all the gene in one cell of a living thing (*Human genome*).
- **Marker:** an indicator or characteristic trait of a disease that facilitates differential diagnosis (*A marker for hepatitis*).
- **Screening:** medical tests that are done on a lot of people to make sure that they do not have a particular disease (*Screening for breast cancer*).

- **Drug (to):** drogare, dare, prendere farmaci.

- **Challenge:** sfida, provocazione.
- **Driver gene mutation:** mutazione pilota del gene.
- **Highlight (to):** evidenziare, sottolineare, mettere in luce.
- **Pathway:** sentiero, tracciato, via (metabolica).
- **Resequencing methods:** metodi per risequenziare un gene.
- **Schedule:** piano, tabella, scala.
- **Throughput:** produttività, capacità di trattamento.

Exercise 4

Decide which statements are true (T) or false (F).

		T	F
1.	The admission is free.		
2.	People attending the lecture do not need to be registered.		
3.	You can't get your registration before the 24th of May.		
4.	Students from the University of Manchester can attend the lecture without any registration.		
5.	ICON employees can't attend the lecture.		
6.	There is a general increasing understanding of causes and progression of cancer diseases.		
7.	The lecture discussion is also about the consideration, validation and prioritization of new molecular targets.		
8.	There are new emerging treatments.		
9.	The "pharmacological audit trail" can be made on a biomarker basis.		
10.	Pharmaceutical companies are supposed to have a changing role in future challenges for cancer drugging.		

Exercise 5

Give the Italian for.

1. The discovery of molecularly targeted small molecule cancer drugs
....
2. ... responsible for the initiation and malignant progression of cancer
....
3. ... survival rates in the major solid tumours have not been extended dramatically
....
4. ... new mechanism-based molecular therapeutics
....
5. ... cancer drugs are leading the way in the development of personalised molecular medicines
....
6. Future challenges for drugging the cancer genome will be highlighted
....

Exercise 6

Translate the fragments in italics into English.

1. We are currently living an incredibily exciting and productive era for *la scoperta e lo sviluppo di farmaci anticancro.*

   ...

2. The molecular targets *degli attuali progetti di scoperta di farmaci* now reflects our increasing, *benché ancora incompleta, comprensione* of the genes and *i percorsi che sono responsabili* for the initiation and malignant progression of cancer.

   ...

3. *In questa conferenza avrò lo scopo di* capture the sense of excitement and describe the opportunities *e sfide nella scoperta e nella concezione* of molecularly targeted small molecule cancer drugs.

   ...

4. *Le tecnologie ad alta produttività stanno accelerando* the rate of cancer gene discovery, but also *rivelando un alto livello di complessità.*

   ...

5. The new treatments *che stanno emergendo nell'ultima decade* are beginning to reflect the success of new mechanism-based molecular therapeutics that act on cancer-causing targets *e hanno tratto beneficio dalle innovazioni tecnologiche nella progettazione dei farmaci.*

   ...

UNIT 11

INTRODUCTION TO CHEMISTRY

CHEMISTRY: THE CENTRAL SCIENCE

Chemistry is often called the "central science" because it connects other sciences, such as physics, material science, nanotechnology, biology, pharmacy, bioinformatics, and geology. These connections are formed through various sub-disciplines that utilize concepts from multiple scientific disciplines. For example, physical chemistry involves applying the principles of physics to materials at the atomic and molecular level. The precise nature of the theoretical connection that chemistry (along with the other so-called special sciences) has with physics is a matter of research in philosophy of science.

Chemistry pertains to the interactions of matter. These interactions may be between two material substances or between matter and energy, especially in conjunction with the First Law of Thermodynamics. Traditional chemistry involves interactions between substances in chemical reactions, where one or more substances become one or more other substances. Sometimes these reactions are driven by energetic (enthalpic) considerations, such as when two highly energetic substances such as elemental hydrogen and oxygen react to form the less energetic substance water. Chemists often use reaction equations to summarize a specific reaction. The chemical reaction between hydrogen and oxygen is shown in the following equation:

$$2H_2 + O_2 \rightarrow 2H_2O$$

The number of atoms on the left and the right of the arrow is always equal in chemical reactions. Other reactions are driven primarily by entropy, which, simply stated, is a measure of disorder. Chemical reactions may be facilitated by a catalyst, which is generally another chemical substance present within the reaction media but unconsumed (such as sulphuric acid catalyzing the electrolysis of water) or a non-material phenomenon (such as electromagnetic radiation in photochemical reactions). Traditional chemistry also deals with the analysis of chemicals both in and apart from a reaction, as in spectroscopy.

All ordinary matter consists of atoms or the subatomic components that make up atoms; protons, electrons and neutrons. Atoms may be combined to produce more complex forms of matter such as ions, molecules or crystals. The structure of the world we commonly experience and the properties of the matter we commonly interact with are determined by properties of chemical substances and their interactions. Steel is harder than iron because its atoms are bound together in a more rigid crystalline lattice. Wood burns or undergoes rapid oxidation because it can react spontaneously with oxygen in a chemical reaction above a certain temperature. Sugar and salt dissolve in water because their molecular/ionic properties allow this.

Substances tend to be classified in terms of their energy or phase as well as their chemical compositions. The three phases of matter at low energy are Solid, Liquid and Gas. Solids have fixed structures at room temperature, which can resist gravity and other weak forces attempting to rearrange them, due to their tight bonds. Liquids have limited bonds, with no structure and flow with gravity. Gases have no bonds and act as free particles. Another way to view the three phases is by volume and shape: roughly speaking, solids have fixed volume and shape, liquids have fixed volume but no fixed shape, and gases have neither fixed volume nor fixed shape.

Water (H_2O) is a liquid at room temperature because its molecules are bound by intermolecular forces called Hydrogen bonds. Thus, the forces between the molecules are so large that the energy at room temperature is not high enough to break them. Hydrogen sulphide (H_2S) on the other hand is a gas at room temperature and standard pressure, as its molecules are bound by weaker dipole-dipole interactions. The hydrogen bonds in water have enough energy to keep the water molecules from separating from each other but not from sliding around, making it a liquid at temperatures between 0 °C and 100 °C at sea level. Lowering the temperature or energy further, allows for a tighter organization to form, creating a solid, and releasing energy. Increasing the energy will melt the ice although the temperature will not change until all the ice is melted. Increasing the temperature of the water will eventually cause boiling when there is enough energy to overcome the polar attractions between individual water molecules (100 °C at 1 atmosphere of pressure), allowing the H_2O molecules to disperse enough to be a gas. Note that in each case there is energy required to overcome the intermolecular attractions and thus allow the molecules to move away from each other.

First Law of Thermodynamics

The first law of thermodynamics is often called the Law of Conservation of Energy. This law suggests that energy can be transferred from one system to another in many forms. Also, it cannot be created or destroyed. Thus, the total amount of energy available in the Universe is constant. Einstein's famous equation (written below) describes the relationship between energy and matter:

$$E = mc^2.$$

In the equation above, energy (E) is equal to matter (m) times the square of a constant (c). Einstein suggested that energy and matter are interchangeable. His equation also suggests that the quantity of energy and matter in the Universe is fixed.

Scientists who study chemistry are known as chemists. Most chemists specialize in one or more sub-disciplines. The chemistry taught at the high school or early college level is often called "general chemistry" and is intended to be an introduction to a wide variety of fundamental concepts and to give the student the tools to continue on to more advanced subjects. Many concepts presented at this level are often incomplete and technically inaccurate, yet they are of extraordinary utility. Chemists regularly use these simple, elegant tools and explanations in their work because they have been proven to accurately model a very wide array of chemical reactivity, are generally sufficient, and more precise solutions may be prohibitively difficult to obtain.

WORD FILE

- **Biology:** the scientific study of living things.
- **Catalyst:** a substance which, without itself changing, quickens chemical processes.
- **Chemistry:** the science which studies the substances which make up the earth, universe, and living things how these substances combine with each other, and how they behave under different conditions.
- **Crystal:** a small regular shape that some chemicals make when they become solid.
- **Dipole:** a particle or object bearing opposite partial charges.

- **Electrolysis:** the separation of a liquid into its chemical parts by passing electricity through it from an anode to a cathode.
- **Electron:** negatively charged subatomic particle.
- **Energy:** the power from electricity, gas, coal, atom etc. that is used to make machines work and to make heat and light.
- **Entropy:** a measure of the degree of disorder in a system, which takes into account the fact that disorder naturally increases with the passage of time.
- **Equation:** a statement that two quantities are equal.
- **Geology:** the study of materials such as soil, rocks etc. which make up the Earth.
- **Hydrogen:** a gas that is a simple substance without colour or smell, is lighter than air and burns very easily.
- **Ion:** an atom which has been given (+) positive or (-) negative charge by the taking away or addition of an electron.
- **Iron:** name of the element Fe.
- **Matter:** the physical material of which everything that we can see or touch is made.
- **Molecule:** the smallest unit into which a substance can be divided without losing its own chemical nature, consisting usually of two or more atoms.
- **Nanotechnology:** a branch of technology applied to extremely small objects.
- **Neutron:** a subatomic particle that carries no electricity and that together with the proton forms the nucleus of an atom.
- **Oxygen:** a gas present in the air that is a simple substance, without colour, taste or smell and is necessary for all forms of life on Earth.
- **Phenomenon:** (pl. phenomena) a fact or event that exists and can be experienced by the senses, especially one that is unusual and of scientific interest.
- **Proton:** a very small piece of matter that carries positive electricity and that together with the neutron forms the nucleus.
- **Spectroscopy:** the use of a spectroscope.
- **Steel:** a metal consisting of iron in a hard strong form containing some carbon and sometimes other metals.
- **Sulfide (sulphide):** a compound made of sulphur and another element.

- **Attempt (to):** tentare, provare, cercare di.
- **Bind (to), bound, bound:** legare, obbligare, costringere.
- **Bond:** legame, vincolo.
- **Burn (to), burnt, burnt:** bruciare.
- **Due to:** a causa di, grazie a, per.
- **Flow (to):** scorrere, fluire.
- **Hard:** duro, rigido.
- **Increase (to):** aumentare, far salire. *Decrease:* diminuire
- **Melt (to):** sciogliere (*The snow melted into water*).
- **On the other hand:** d'altro canto.
- **Overcome (to):** superare, sopraffare, vincere.
- **Rearrange (to):** risistemare, ridisporre.
- **Room temperature:** temperature ambiente.
- **Rough:** ruvido. *Roughly speaking:* esprimendosi impropriamente.
- **Sea level:** livello del mare.
- **Tight:** stretto, ma anche forte.
- **Tools:** attrezzi.
- **Undergo (to):** sopportare, essere sottoposti a, subire.
- **Weak:** debole, fievole.

Exercise 1

Match the words from the left with the ones from the right.

1. steel	a. scorrere
2. overcome	b. legame
3. rough	c. ruvido
4. tight	d. superare
5. flow	e. acciaio
6. melt	f. debole
7. bond	g. stretto
8. weak	h. sciogliere

Exercise 2

Give the English for the following.

1. Livello del mare. ....
2. D'altro canto. ....
3. A causa di. ....
4. Bruciare. ....
5. Ferro. ....
6. Acciaio. ....
7. Temperatura ambiente. ....
8. Legare. ....
9. Freccia. ....
10. Solfato. ....

Exercise 3

Fill in the gaps with a suitable word from the passage.

1. Chemistry pertains to the interactions of .... These .... may be between two material substances or between matter and ...., especially in conjunction with the First .... of Thermodynamics.
2. Chemists often use reaction equations to .... a specific reaction. The chemical reaction between hydrogen and oxygen is .... in the following ....: $2H_2 + O_2 \rightarrow 2H_2O$.
3. All ordinary matter .... of atoms or the subatomic components that .... atoms; protons, electrons and neutrons. Atoms may .... to produce more complex forms of matter .... ions, molecules or crystals. The .... of the world we commonly experience and the properties of the .... we commonly interact with are determined by .... of chemical substances and their interactions.

4. Substances tend to .... in terms of their energy or phase as .... as their chemical compositions. The three phases of matter at low energy are Solid, Liquid and Gas. Solids have fixed structures at .... temperature which can resist .... and other .... forces attempting to rearrange them, ... their tight bonds. Liquids have limited ...., with no structure and flow with gravity. Gases have .... bonds and act .... free particles.
5. Increasing the .... of the water will eventually cause .... when there is enough energy to .... the polar .... between individual water molecules (100 °C at 1 atmosphere of pressure), ... the H_2O molecules to disperse .... to be a gas.

Exercise 4

Translate the fragments in italics into English.

1. The number of the atoms *a sinistra e a destra* of the arrow is always equal in chemical reactions.

   ....

   ....

2. All ordinary matter *consistono* in atoms or subatomic components *che formano gli atomi.*

   ....

   ....

3. Atoms may be combined to produce *forme più complesse* of matter *come gli ioni, le molecole o i cristalli.*

   ....

   ....

4. Steel is *più resistente del ferro* because its atoms are bound *insieme in un più rigido* crystalline lattice.

   ....

   ....

5. *I solidi* have fixed structures at room temperature *che possono* resist gravity and other weak forces *cercando* to rearrange them, *grazie ai loro forti* bonds.

   ....

   ....

6. *Le forze* between the molecules are *così ampie che* the energy at room temperature is not *abbastanza alta* to break them.

   ....

   ....

7. Increasing the energy *scioglierà il ghiaccio* although the temperature *non cambierà fino a quando* all the ice *sarà sciolto.*

   ....

   ....

8. *Molti concetti* presented at this level are often *incompleti e tecnicamente imprecisi, tuttavia* they are of extraordinary utility.

....

....

Exercise 5

Rewrite the following sentences.

1. Wood burns because it can react spontaneously with oxygen in a chemical reaction above a certain temperature.

....

....

2. Water (H_2O) is a liquid at room temperature because its molecules are bound by intermolecular forces called Hydrogen bonds.

....

....

....

3. Increasing the temperature of the water will eventually cause boiling when there is enough energy to overcome the polar attractions between individual water molecules.

....

....

....

4. The chemistry taught at the high school or early college level is often called "general chemistry" and is intended to be an introduction to a wide variety of fundamental concepts and to give the student the tools to continue on to more advanced subjects.

....

....

....

Exercise 6

Answer the following questions.

1. Which are the other sciences connected to chemistry?

....

2. Which kind of interactions does chemistry involve?

....

3. What does a catalyst do?

....

4. Why is steel harder than iron?

....

5. Why is water liquid at room temperature?

....

PREDICTING CHEMICAL EFFECTS (BASED ON UNKNOWN RESPONSES)

Structure-Activity Relationship (SAR) is a means by which the effect of a drug or toxic chemical on an animal, plant, or the environment can be related to its molecular structure. This type of relationship may be assessed by considering a series of molecules, each with a slightly different structure, then noting the difference in biological activity associated with each structural variation. Alternatively, it may be possible to assess a large body of data using intelligent tools such as neural networks to try to establish relationships between structures and activity.
Ideally, such relationships can be characterized mathematically as Quantitative Structure Activity Relationships (QSAR), in which some degree of predictive capability is present. This field of science therefore combines mathematics and chemistry and is called computational chemistry. Scientists use this information to predict where a chemical goes in the environment or the toxicity of a chemical. Since QSARs are equations that help to predict fate or effect values from chemical structure, they are quick and inexpensive to use.
The QSAR paradigm is based on the assumption that there is an underlying relationship between molecular structure and biological activity. Also it is assumed that the multivariate physicochemical description of the set of compounds reveal these analogies. All physical, chemical, and biological properties of a chemical substance can be computed from its molecular structure, encoded in a numerical form with the aid of various descriptors. Indeed QSAR is based in the well-known similarity principle, which states that similar compounds have similar activities. In addition, besides from the aforementioned similarity principle also the neighbourhood principle holds. This principle states that, in principle, molecules located in the same region of the descriptor space present similar activity.

Pay attention

Means ➢ mezzi
– mantiene la "s" anche al singolare.

By means: per mezzo di.
By all means: con ogni mezzo possibile.
The undergound is a convenient means of transport.
By all means: certamente. *By no means:* in nessun modo.

BUFFER SOLUTIONS

A buffer solution is made by mixing a buffer agent's acid form (HA) with its conjugate base (A^-) in water. Once a balance exists between HA and A^-, any other acids or bases added to the buffer solution will be neutralized when they turn a portion of the buffer agent into either the HA or A^- form. The change in the buffer agent initially causes little change in the buffer solution's pH. As the proportion of a buffer agent's HA and A^- changes due to the addition of other acids and bases, the buffering capacity of the solution decreases. Eventually, a buffer agent can be used up to the point where it can no longer significantly resist pH changes, meaning it is no longer useful as a buffer solution.
Buffer solutions and buffer agents are extremely common. The detergent borax, for instance, can be used to make a simple buffer solution. Many traditional antacid tablets are, in fact, buffer

agents that work within the human body. Buffered aspirin is aspirin that has been treated with a buffering agent to help reduce pH changes to the aspirin when it is exposed to stomach acid. pH probes are protected from damage by being stored in buffer solutions.

In the human body, buffer agents play a vital role in both respiration and maintaining the body's pH level. One of the most important buffer agents in humans is bicarbonate. When carbon dioxide (CO_2) mixes with water (H_2O), carbonic acid is formed (H_2CO_3). Bicarbonate (HCO_3^-) is a dissociation of carbonic acid. Carbonic acid and bicarbonate form an equilibrium in the blood that helps the body adjust to pH changes.

Just like a buffer solution, the bicarbonate/carbonic acid equilibrium will no longer resist pH changes if their proportions are significantly altered. Excesses of carbonic acid are adjusted by forming carbon dioxide through the removal of water from carbonic acid; the carbon dioxide is then exhaled. Excessive amounts of bicarbonate can be reduced by inhaling more carbon dioxide, which is then changed into carbonic acid.

Buffer Systems in Blood

The body maintains the pH of blood at around 7.4. If the pH level changes just a few tenths of a pH unit, serious health consequences can result. A decrease in blood pH is called acidosis, an increase is called alkalosis. Three different buffer systems exist in blood, the bicarbonate buffer and the phosphate buffer are composed of "simple" chemicals. In addition the carbonyl groups (-COOH) and the amide group (-NH2) present on proteins allow some of these to act as buffers.

Exercise 7

Answer the following questions.

1. What is a buffer solution made from?

   ....

   ....

2. When does the buffering capacity of the solution decrease?

   ....

   ....

3. What does the "buffered aspirin" consist of?

   ....

   ....

4. What is the role of the buffering agents in the human body?

   ....

   ....

5. Give the name of one of the most important buffer agent in the human body?

   ....

   ....

6. What happens when there are excesses of carbonic acid?

   ....

   ....

Exercise 8

Read again the previous passages and fill in the blanks.

Ideally, such relationships .... characterized mathematically as Quantitative Structure Activity Relationships (QSAR), ... some degree of predictive capability is present. This field of science therefore combines mathematics and chemistry and .... called computational chemistry. Scientists use this information to predict .... a chemical goes in the environment or the toxicity of a chemical. Since QSARs are equations .... help to predict fate or effect values from chemical structure, they are quick and inexpensive to use.

A buffer solution .... by mixing a buffer agent's acid form (HA) with its conjugate base (A-) in water. Once a balance exists between HA and A-, any other acids or bases added to the buffer solution .... neutralized when they turn a portion of the buffer agent into .... the HA .... A- form. The change in the buffer agent initially causes little change in the buffer solution's pH. As the proportion of a buffer agent's HA and A- changes .... the addition of other acids and bases, the buffering capacity of the solution decreases. Eventually, a buffer agent .... be used up to the point where it can no longer significantly resist pH changes, meaning it is .... useful as a buffer solution.

LAB GLOSSARY

- **Buchner funnel:** imbuto filtrante.
- **Burette:** buretta.
- **Crucible:** crogiolo.
- **Dessicator:** essiccatore.
- **Droppe:** contagocce.
- **Graham reflux condenser:** condensatore a ricadere.
- **Incubator:** incubatore.
- **Laminar flow hood:** cappa a flusso laminare.
- **Magnetic stirrer:** agitatore magnetico.
- **Melting point apparatus:** apparato per la determinazione del punto di fusione.
- **Microscope slide:** vetrino per microscopia.
- **Mortar and pestle:** mortaio e pestello.
- **PH meter:** piaccametro.
- **Rotating evaporator:** evaporatore rotante.
- **Scalpel:** bisturi.
- **Serological pipette:** pipetta graduata sterile.
- **Spectrophotometer:** spettrofotometro.
- **Stir rod:** agitatore.
- **Stopper:** tappo.
- **Test tube:** provetta.
- **Thin layer chromatography:** (TLC) cromatografia su strato sottile.
- **Tweezer:** pinzetta.
- **Watch glass:** vetro d'orologio.

UNIT 12

NATURAL REMEDIES

HERBAL MEDICINE

Herbal medicine, also called botanical medicine or phytomedicine, refers to the use of any plant's seeds, berries, roots, leaves, bark, or flowers for medicinal purposes. Long practiced outside of conventional medicine, herbalism is becoming more common as up-dated researches showed its value in the treatment and prevention of disease.

What is the History of Herbal Medicine?

Plants had been used for medicinal purposes long before recorded history. For example, ancient African and Native American used herbs in their healing rituals, while others developed traditional medical systems (e.g., Ayurveda and Traditional Chinese Medicine) in which herbal therapies were used systematically. Scientists found that people in different parts of the globe tended to use the same or similar plants for the same purposes.

In the early 19th century, when methods of chemical analysis first became available, scientists began extracting and modifying the active ingredients from plants. Later, chemists began making their own version of plant compounds, beginning the transition from raw herbs to synthetic pharmaceuticals. Over time, the use of herbal medicines declined in favor of pharmaceuticals. Recently, the World Health Organization estimated that 80% of people worldwide rely on herbal medicines for some aspect of their primary healthcare. In the last twenty years in the United States, increasing public dissatisfaction with the cost of prescription medications, combined with an interest in returning to natural or organic remedies, has led to an increase in the use of herbal medicines. In Germany, roughly 600 to 700 plant-based medicines are available and are prescribed by approximately 70% of German physicians.

Ayurveda is a system of traditional medicine native to the Indian Subcontinent and practiced in other parts of the world as a form of alternative medicine.
Evolving throughout its history, Ayurveda remains an influential system of medicine in South Asia. Ayurveda is considered to be a form of complementary and alternative medicine (CAM) within the western world, where several of its methods, such as the use of herbs, massage, and Yoga as exercise or alternative medicine, are applied on their own as a form of CAM treatment.

How Do Herbs Work?

For most herbs, the specific ingredient that causes a therapeutic effect is not known. Whole herbs contain many ingredients (phytocomplex), and it is likely that they work together to produce the desired medicinal effect. Many factors affect how effective an herb will be. For example, the type of environment (climate, bugs, soil quality) in which a plant grew will affect its components, as will how and when it was harvested and processed.

How Are Herbs Used?

For the reasons described in the previous section, herbalists prefer using whole plants rather than extracting single components from them. Whole plant extracts have many components. These components work together to produce therapeutic effects and also to lessen the chances of side effects from any one component. Several herbs are often used together to enhance effectiveness and synergistic actions and to reduce toxicity. Herbalists must take many things into account when prescribing herbs. For example, the species and variety of the plant, the plant's habitat, how it was stored and processed, and whether or not there are contaminants.

What Happens during a Visit to an Herbalist?

When you visit an herbalist, the treatment goals are often more broad than stopping a single complaint. Herbalists aim to correct imbalances, resolve patterns of dysfunction, and treat the underlying cause of your complaint. Specific symptoms may also be treated if necessary.

A session with an herbalist typically lasts one hour. You may be physically examined and asked about your medical history and your general well-being (that is, how well you sleep, what you eat, if you have a good appetite, good digestion and elimination, how often you exercise, and what you do to relax). The herbalist might recommend one or more herbs, dietary changes, and lifestyle modifications. Because herbal medicines are slower acting than pharmaceuticals, you might be asked to return for a follow-up in two to four weeks.

Who Is Using Herbal Medicine?

Nearly one-third of Americans use herbs and it is estimated that in 1998 alone $4 billion was spent on herbal products in this country. Unfortunately, a recent study in the *New England Journal of Medicine* indicated that nearly 70% of individuals taking herbal medicines (the majority of which were well educated and had a higher-than-average income) were reluctant to reveal their use of complementary and alternative medicine to their doctors. Because herbal medicines contain a combination of chemicals, each with a specific action, many are capable of eliciting complex physiological responses – some of which may create unwanted or unexpected results when combined with conventional drugs. Be sure to consult your doctor before trying any herbal products.

How Is Herbal Medicine Sold in Stores?

The herbs available in most stores come in several different forms: teas, syrups, oils, liquid extracts, tinctures, and dry extracts (pills or capsules). Teas are simply dried herbs left to soak for a few minutes in boiling water. Syrups, made from concentrated extracts and added to sweet-tasting preparations, are frequently used for sore throats and coughs. Oils are extracted from plants and often used as rubs for massage, either alone or as part of an ointment or cream. Tinctures and liquid extracts are solvents (usually water, alcohol, or glycerol) that contain the active ingredients of the herbs. Tinctures are typically a 1:5 or 1:10 concentration, meaning that one part of the herbal material is prepared with five to ten parts (by weight) of the liquid. Liquid extracts are more concentrated than tinctures and are typically a 1:1 concentration. A dry extract form is the most concentrated form of an herbal product (typically 2:1 to 8:1) and is sold as a tablet, capsule, or lozenge.

Currently, no organization or government body regulates the manufacture or certifies the labeling of herbal preparations. This means you can't be sure that the amount of the herb contained in the bottle, or even from dose to dose, is the same as what is stated on the label. Some herbal preparations are standardized, meaning that the preparation is *guaranteed* to contain a specific amount of one active ingredient of the herb. However, it is still important to ask companies that are making standardized herbal products the basis for their product's guarantee. If consumers insist on an answer to this question, manufacturers of these herbal products may begin to implement more quality control processes, like microscopic, chemical, and biological analyses. Again, it is important to consult your doctor or an expert in herbal medicine for the recommended doses of any herbal products you are considering.

The American Herbalists Guild
The American Herbalists Guild was founded in 1989 as a non-profit, educational organization to represent the goals and voices of herbalists specializing in the medicinal use of plants. Its primary goal is to promote a high level of professionalism and education in the study and practice of therapeutic herbalism.
For more information:
www.americanherbalistsguild.com
www.naturopathic.org

Are there Experts in Herbal Medicine?

Herbalists, chiropractors, naturopathic physicians, and practitioners of Traditional Chinese Medicine all use herbs to treat illness. Naturopathic physicians believe that the body is continually striving for balance and that natural therapies can be used to support this process. They are trained in four-year, postgraduate institutions that combine courses in conventional medical science (such as pathology, microbiology, pharmacology, and surgery) with clinical training in herbal medicine, homeopathy, nutrition, and lifestyle counseling.

What is the Future of Herbal Medicine?

Although a renaissance is occurring in herbal medicine in the United States, the FDA still classifies herbs as dietary supplements and forbids manufacturers to claim that their products are able to treat or prevent specific diseases. In some countries in Europe, however, herbs are classified as drugs and are regulated. The German Commission E, an expert medical panel, actively researches their safety and effectiveness.

[University of Maryland www.umm.edu/altmed/articles/herbal.medicine, adapted from]

WORD FILE

- **Chiropractor:** some who treats physical problems by pressing on and moving the bones in someone's back and joints.
- **Herbalist:** someone who grows, sells, or uses herbs to treat illness. (*An herbalist:* perché in American English la parola *herbs* può essere considerata iniziante con "h" muta).

- **Bug:** cimice (qui insetti generico). Agente infettivo (colloquiale).
- **Cough:** tosse.
- **Dietary supplement:** integratore alimentare.
- **Enhance (to):** migliorare, rafforzare.
- **Environment:** ambiente.
- **Harvest:** raccolto.
- **Lozenge:** pasticca (fatta a losanga).
- **Raw:** grezzo. *Raw materials:* materie prime.
- **Rely on (to):** contare su.
- **Rub:** frizione, massaggio.
- **Soak (to):** immergere, immergersi.
- **Sore throat:** mal di gola.
- **Strive (to):** lottare, battersi, sforzarsi.
- **Underlying:** sottostante.
- **Up-dated:** aggiornato.

Exercise 1

Give a definition using your own words.

1. Herbalist. ....
2. Naturopathic physician. ....

Exercise 2

Answer the following questions.

1. What happens during a session with an herbalist?

   ....

   ....

2. Give reasons for the increase in the use of herbal remedies

   ....

   ....

Exercise 3

Decide which statements are true (T) or false (F).

		T	F
1.	Herbal medicines are faster acting than pharmaceuticals.	■	■
2.	A large majority of people taking herbal medicines are reluctant to speak about their use to their doctors.	■	■
3.	Syrups are made from dried herbs.	■	■
4.	In tinctures one part of the herbal material is prepared with five to 10 parts of the liquid.	■	■
5.	Herbal preparations are certified as much as their labeling is concerned.	■	■
6.	The type of environment can affect the effectiveness of a plant.	■	■
7.	Herbal medicines are classified as dietary supplements.	■	■
8.	The most concentrated form of an herbal product is the dry form.	■	■

WHAT IS HERBAL MEDICINE GOOD FOR?

Herbalists treat many conditions such as asthma, eczema, premenstrual syndrome, rheumatoid arthritis, migraine, menopausal symptoms, chronic fatigue, and irritable bowel syndrome, among others. Herbal preparations are best taken under the guidance of a trained professional. Be sure to consult with your doctor or an herbalist before self-treating. Some common herbs and their uses are discussed below.

- **Ginkgo (*Ginkgo biloba*)**, particularly a standardized extract known as EGb 761, appears to produce improvements in awareness, judgment, and social function in people with Alzheimer's disease and dementia. In a year-long study of 309 people with Alzheimer's disease, those taking EGb 761 consistently improved while those on placebo worsened.
- **Kava kava (*Piper methysticum*)** has become popular as a treatment for anxiety, but recent reports have traced liver damage to enough people who have used kava that the US FDA has

issued a warning regarding its use and other countries, such as Germany and Canada, have taken kava off of the market.

- **St. John's wort** *(Hypericum perforatum)* is well known for its antidepressant effects, and an analysis of 27 studies involving more than 2,000 people confirmed that the herb is an effective treatment for mild to moderate depression.
- **Valerian** *(Valeriana officinalis)* has had a long tradition as a sleep-inducing agent, with the added benefit of producing no hangover feeling the next day.
- **Echinacea** (from ***Echinacea purpurea*** and other ***Echinacea*** species) may bolster immunity. In a study of 160 volunteers with flu-like symptoms, echinacea extract reduced both the frequency and severity of cold symptoms.

Warning

Used correctly, many herbs are considered safer than conventional medications, but because they are unregulated, herbal products are often mislabeled and may contain undeclared additives and adulterants. Some herbs are associated with allergic reactions or interact with conventional drugs. Self-prescribing herbal products will increase your risk, so it is important to consult your doctor and an herbalist before taking herbal medicines. Some examples of adverse reactions from certain popular herbs are described below.

- **St. John's wort** causes sensitivity to the sun's ultraviolet rays, and may cause an allergic reaction, stomach upset, fatigue, and restlessness. Studies show that St. John's wort also interferes with the effectiveness of many drugs, including warfarin (an anticoagulant), protease inhibitors for HIV, possibly birth control pills, and many other medications. In addition, St. John's wort must not be taken with anti-depressant medication. The Food and Drug Administration (FDA) has issued a public health advisory concerning many of these interactions.
- **Kava kava** and **echinacea** have both been linked to liver toxicity. Again, kava has been taken off the market in several countries because of the liver toxicity.
- **Valerian** may cause oversedation, and in some people it may even have the unexpected effect of overstimulating instead of sedating.
- **Feverfew** (***Tanacetum parthenium***) may cause agitation.

Bleeding time may be altered with the use of **garlic, ginkgo, feverfew, ginger** (***Zingiber officinalis***) and **ginseng.**

[University of Maryland www.umm.edu/altmed/articles/herbal.medicine, adapted from]

WORD FILE

- **Hangover:** pain in your head and a feeling of sickness like the one you get the day after you have drunk too much alcohol.

- **Bark:** corteccia.
- **Berry:** bacca.
- **Bolster (to):** sostenere.
- **Bowel:** intestino.
- **Feverfew:** erba amara vera.
- **Garlic:** aglio.
- **Ginger:** zenzero.
- **Kava kava:** kava.
- **Lessen (to):** abbassare, diminuire.
- **Seed:** seme.
- **St John's wort:** iperico.
- **Worsen (to):** peggiorare.

Exercise 4

Fill in the table.

Herbs	Suggested for
Echinacea	
Valerian	
Kava kava	
St. John's wort	
Ginko Biloba	

A dietary supplement, also known as food supplement or nutritional supplement, is a preparation intended to provide nutrients, such as vitamins, minerals, fiber, fatty acids or amino acids, that are missing or are not consumed in sufficient quantity in a person's diet. Some countries define dietary supplements as foods, while in others they are defined as drugs.

Exercise 5

Give the Italian for.

1. Mislabelled. ....
2. Adulterants. ....
3. Conventional drugs. ....
4. Sleep-inducting agent. ....
5. Self-prescribing herbal products. ....
6. Irritable bowel syndrome. ....
7. Counselling. ....
8. Follow-up. ....

TRADITIONAL AND COMPLEMENTARY/ALTERNATIVE MEDICINE (TM/CAM)

TC/CAM are healing resources that encompasses all health systems, modalities, and practices and their accompanying theories and belief, other than those intrinsic to the politically dominant health system, even if the boundaries between TM/CAM and the commonly used medicine of the western world are not always sharp or fixed.
Traditional medicine is becoming more popular throughout the world and up to 80% of people in the developing countries use it as part of primary health care. The situation has given rise to concerns among health practitioners and consumers on the issue of safety, above all, but also on questions of

policy, regulation, evidence, biodiversity and preservation and protection of traditional knowledge. As 80% of the people in Africa use traditional medicine it is necessary to evaluate its safety, efficacy, quality and standardization – as well as to protect the heritage and to preserve the traditional knowledge. In wealthy countries, growing numbers of patients rely on alternative medicine for preventive or palliative care. But problems may arise out of incorrect use of traditional therapies. Traditional or complementary medicine is victim of both uncritical enthusiasts and uninformed sceptics.
The global market for traditional therapies has been steadily growing. In addition to the patient safety issue and the threat to knowledge and biodiversity, there is also the risk that further commercialization through unregulated use will make these therapies unaffordable to many who rely on them as their primary source of health care. For this reason policies on the protection of indigenous or traditional knowledge are necessary.
The correct use and development of TM/CAM requires:

- develop national policies on the evaluation and regulation of TM/CAM practices;
- create a stronger evidence base on the safety, efficacy and quaity of the TM/CAM products and practices;
- ensure availability and affordability of TM/CAM, including essential herbal medicines;
- promote therapeutically sound use of TM/CAM by providers and consumers.

[*Essential Drugs in brief*, by the WHO, adapted from]

NCCAM

The **National Center for Complementary and Alternative Medicine** or **NCCAM**, is a *United States* government agency. NCCAM is dedicated to exploring complementary and alternative healing practices in the context of rigorous science, training complementary and alternative medicine (CAM) researchers, and providing information about CAM.
The NCCAM is one of the 27 institutes and centers that make up the *National Institutes of Health* (NIH) within the *Department of Health and Human Services* of the *federal government of the United States*. The NIH is one of eight agencies under the *Public Health Service* (PHS) in the *Department of Health and Human Services* (DHHS).

NCCAM
NATIONAL CENTER FOR COMPLEMENTARY AND ALTERNATIVE MEDICINE

Exercise 6

Fill in the blanks using words from the box.

• primary source • throughout the world • unaffordable • growing • primary • palliative care • wealthy • health practitioners • to evaluate • issue

Traditional medicine is becoming more popular .... and up to 80% of people in the developing countries use it as part of .... health care. The situation has given rise to concerns among .... and consumers on the issue of safety. As 80% of the people in Africa use traditional medicine it is necessary .... its safety, efficacy, quality and standardization—as well as to protect the heritage and to preserve the traditional knowledge. In .... countries, growing numbers of patients rely on alternative medicine for preventive or .... But problems may arise out of incorrect use of traditional therapies.

The global market for traditional therapies has been steadily .... In addition to the patient safety .... and the threat to knowledge and biodiversity, there is also the risk that further commercialization through unregulated use will make these therapies .... to many who rely on them as their .... of health care.

ABOUT HOMOEOPATHY

A leading medical journal has made a damning attack on homoeopathy, saying it is no better than dummy drugs.

The Lancet says the time for more studies is over and doctors should be bold and honest with patients about homoeopathy's "lack of benefit".

A Swiss-UK review of 110 trials found no convincing evidence the treatment worked any better than a placebo. Advocates of homoeopathy maintained the therapy, which works on the principle of treating like with like, does work: someone with an allergy, for example, who was using homoeopathic medicines would attempt to beat it with an ultra-diluted dose of an agent that would cause the same symptoms.

The row over homeopathy has been raging for years.

In 2002, American illusionist James Randi offered $1m to anyone able to prove, under observed conditions in a laboratory, that homeopathic remedies can really cure people. To date, no-one has passed the preliminary tests.

In 2000, the UK Parliamentary Select Committee on Science and Technology issued a report on complementary and alternative medicine. It reported that "any therapy that makes specific claims for being able to treat specific conditions should have evidence of being able to do this above and beyond the placebo effect".

According to Professor Matthias Egger, from the University of Berne, and Swiss colleagues from Zurich University and a UK team at the University of Bristol, homoeopathy has no such evidence. They compared 110 trials that looked at the effects of homoeopathy versus placebo with 110 trials of conventional medicines for the same medical disorders or diseases.

This included trials for the treatment of asthma, allergies and muscular problems, some large and some small.

For both homoeopathy and conventional medicines, the smaller trials of lower quality showed more beneficial treatment effects than the larger trials.

However, when they looked at only the larger, high-quality trials, they found no convincing evidence that homoeopathy worked any better than placebo.

Professor Egger said: "We acknowledge to prove a negative is impossible. But good large studies of homoeopathy do not show a difference between the placebo and the homoeopathic remedy, whereas in the case of conventional medicines you still see an effect."

He said some people do report feeling better after having homoeopathy. He believes this is down to the whole experience of the therapy, with the homoeopath spending a lot of time and attention on the individual: "It has nothing to do with what is in the little white pill," he said.

[From BBC News, 25 august 2005]

Exercise 7

State which statements are true (T) or false (F).

		T	F
1.	The Lancet states that patients cannot get any benefits from homoeopathy.		
2.	Homoeopathy works on the principle of treating like with like.		
3.	There are evidences that homeopathy can work better than placebos.		
4.	Conventional medicines proved better effects than homeopathic medicines.		
5.	Professor Egger pretends that the favourable effects of homeopathy are due to the way homeopathic physicians treat patients.		

AROMATHERAPY

Essential oils offer a wide variety of health benefits such as physical, mental, emotional and spiritual balance. Aromatherapy encompasses over 9000 years of history that supports, exemplifies and solidifies the therapeutic properties essential oils have to offer. It is also fun and empowering as it put control back in YOUR hands over YOUR health choices.

Aromatherapy Benefits

Essential oils are powerful tool that may alter, shift, change and adjust mood, emotion and physical issues. Aromatherapy has been historically known to help alleviate stress, skin irritations, depression and anxiety. It also helps our pets achieve wellness. All 100% pure essential oils are antibacterial. They vary in other properties such as antiviral, antiseptic, anti-inflammatory and so on.

Quality of Aromatherapy

Why is quality important? Well, it will dictate the level of therapeutic value as well as help reduce your exposure to chemical-based products. It is also important when working to enhance overall health and wellness. For example, you may feel relaxed when smelling a synthetic lavender candle but, the combination of synthetic ingredients may bombard and clog the lymphatic system with toxins rather than assist the body in eliminating toxins.

Olfaction Process

Essential Oils have historically been shown to calm and relax emotions as well as enhance focus, attention and memory. To understand this, first it is best to be familiar with the olfaction process. The nose is a protrusion of the brain. Scent enters the body in less than 1 second and travels to the pituitary and hypothalamus to tell your body how to respond to a situation. It will help to relax or stimulate. This message is then sent to the rest of the body via the nervous system. Scent actually dictates how we taste. It is the only sense that does not have to go through the digestive tract or spinal cord to be processed. It immediately goes to the brain and elicits a response. It is also important to note that Richard Axel and Linda Buck (both from the USA) won the 2004 Nobel Prize in Physiology or Medicine for their discoveries of odorant receptors and their relationship to the organization of the olfactory system.

HOLISM

Holism (from holos, a Greek word meaning all, entire, total) is the idea that all the properties of a given system (physical, biological, chemical, social, economic, mental, linguistic, etc.) cannot be determined or explained by its component parts alone. Instead, the system as a whole determines in an important way how the parts behave. The general principle of holism was concisely summarized by Aristotle in the Metaphysics: "The whole is more than the sum of its parts".

Pay attention

Homoeopathy (British English)

Homeopathy (American English)

Studies

There have been numerous studies done to show that the scent of lavender, when inhaled, affects the beta waves thus reducing stress and promoting calmness. Lavender has been historically used to help Alzheimer patients remain calm, relaxed, stay "here in the moment" longer.

[Text from *More about Aromatherapy*, by: Jennifer Hochell NAHA Director]

What is NAHA?
The National Association for Holistic Aromatherapy is an educational, nonprofit organization dedicated to enhancing public awareness of the benefits of true aromatherapy. NAHA is actively involved with promoting and elevating academic standards in aromatherapy education and practice for the profession. NAHA is also actively involved in furthering the publics perception and knowledge of true aromatherapy and its safe and effective application in everyday life.

Exercise 8

Answer the following questions.

1. Which are the benefits of essential oils?
 ....
2. Which are their properties?
 ....
3. Why did Richard Axel and Linda Buck won a Nobel Prize?
 ....

Exercise 9

Complete.

1. The nose is .... of the brain.
2. Scent enters the body in .... and travels to .... to tell your body ....
3. The sense of smell does not have to go through ....
4. There have been numerous studies to show that the scent of .... affects the .... calmness.
5. You may .... relaxed when .... a synthetic lavander candle.

WORD FILE

- **Perfume:** a liquid with a pleasant smell that people put on their skin or clothing to make themselves smell nice.
- **Scent:** a pleasant smell that something has.

- **Clog (to):** intasare, ostruire.
- **Mood:** stato d'animo.
- **Sense of smell:** odorato.
- **Shift (to):** trasferire, mutare.

UNIT 13

HERBAL DRUGS

ALOE VERA

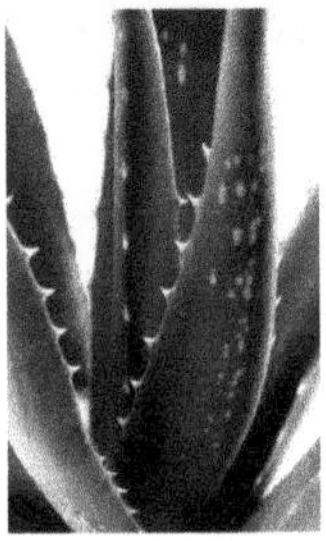

Aloe vera's use can be traced back 6.000 years to early Egyptian civilization, where the plant was depicted on stone carvings. Known as the "plant of immortality," aloe was presented as a burial gift to deceased pharaohs.
Common Names: aloe vera, aloe, burn plant, lily of the desert, elephant's gall.
Latin Names: *Aloe vera, Aloe barbadensis.*

What It Is Used For

Traditionally, aloe was used topically to heal wounds and for various skin conditions, and orally as a laxative. Today, in addition to traditional uses, people take aloe orally to treat a variety of conditions, including diabetes, asthma, epilepsy, and osteoarthritis. People use aloe topically for osteoarthritis, burns, and sunburns.
Aloe vera gel can be found in hundreds of skin products, including lotions and sunblocks.
The Food and Drug Administration (FDA) has approved aloe vera as a natural food flavoring.

How It Is Used

Aloe leaves contain a clear gel that is often used as a topical ointment.
The green part of the leaf that surrounds the gel can be used to produce a juice or a dried substance (called latex) that is taken by mouth.

What the Science Says

Aloe latex contains strong laxative compounds. Products made with various components of aloe (aloin, aloe-emodin, and barbaloin) were at one time regulated by the FDA as oral over-the-counter (OTC) laxatives. In 2002, the FDA required that all OTC aloe laxative products be removed from the US market or reformulated because the companies that manufactured them did not provide the necessary safety data.
Early studies show that topical aloe gel may help heal burns and abrasions. One study, however, showed that aloe gel inhibits healing of deep surgical wounds. Aloe gel does not prevent burns from radiation therapy.
There is not enough scientific evidence to support aloe vera for any of its other uses.

Side Effects and Cautions

Use of topical aloe vera is not associated with significant side effects.

- Abdominal cramps and diarrhea have been reported with oral use of aloe vera.
- Diarrhea, caused by the laxative effect of oral aloe vera, can decrease the absorption of many drugs.
- People with diabetes who use glucose-lowering medication should be cautious if also taking aloe by mouth because preliminary studies suggest aloe may lower blood glucose levels.

BILBERRY

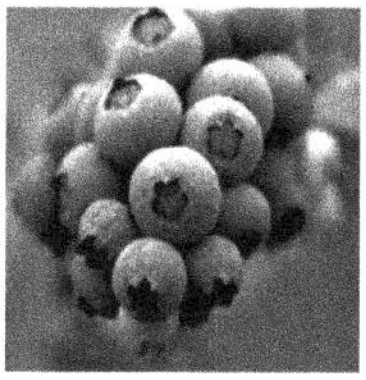

Bilberry is a relative of the blueberry, and its fruit is commonly used to make pies and jams. Bilberry grows in North America, Europe, and northern Asia.
Common Names: European blueberry, whortleberry, huckleberry.
Latin Names: *Vaccinium myrtillus.*

What It Is Used For
Bilberry has been used for nearly 1,000 years in traditional European medicine.
Historically, bilberry fruit was used to treat diarrhea, scurvy, and other conditions.
Today, the fruit is used to treat diarrhea, menstrual cramps, eye problems, varicose veins, venous insufficiency (poor blood flow to the heart), and other circulatory problems.
Bilberry leaf is used for entirely different conditions, including diabetes.

How It Is Used
The fruit of the bilberry plant can be eaten or made into extracts. Similarly, the leaves of the bilberry plant can be made into extracts or used to make teas.

What the Science Says
Some claim that bilberry fruit improves night vision, but clinical studies have not shown this to be true.
There is not enough scientific evidence to support the use of bilberry fruit or leaf for any other health conditions.
NCCAM has not yet funded any research on bilberry.

Side Effects and Cautions
Bilberry fruit is considered safe. However, high doses of bilberry leaf or leaf extract are considered unsafe; animal studies have shown high doses to be toxic.

ASIAN GINSENG

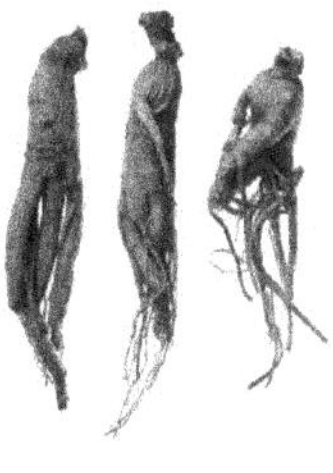

Asian ginseng is native to China and Korea and has been used in various systems of medicine for many centuries. Asian ginseng is one of several types of true ginseng (another is American ginseng, *Panax quinquefolius*). An herb called Siberian ginseng or eleuthero (*Eleutherococcus senticosus*) is not a true ginseng.
Common Names: Asian ginseng, ginseng, Chinese ginseng, Korean ginseng, Asiatic ginseng.
Latin Name: *Panax ginseng.*

What It Is Used For
Treatment claims for Asian ginseng are numerous and include the use of the herb to support overall health and boost the immune system. Traditional and modern uses of ginseng include:

- Improving the health of people recovering from illness;
- Increasing a sense of well-being and stamina, and improving both mental and physical performance;
- Treating erectile dysfunction, hepatitis C, and symptoms related to menopause;
- Lowering blood glucose and controlling blood pressure.

How It Is Used

The root of Asian ginseng contains active chemical components called ginsenosides (or panaxosides) that are thought to be responsible for the herb's medicinal properties. The root is dried and used to make tablets or capsules, extracts, and teas, as well as creams or other preparations for external use.

What the Science Says

Some studies have shown that Asian ginseng may lower blood glucose. Other studies indicate possible beneficial effects on immune function.

To date, research results on Asian ginseng are not conclusive enough to prove health claims associated with the herb. Only a handful of large clinical trials on Asian ginseng have been conducted. Most studies have been small or have had flaws in design and reporting. Some claims for health benefits have been based only on studies conducted in animals.

NCCAM is supporting research studies to better understand the use of Asian ginseng. NCCAM is studying how Asian ginseng interacts with other herbs and drugs and exploring its potential to treat chronic lung infection, impaired glucose tolerance, and Alzheimer's disease.

Side Effects and Cautions

When taken by mouth, ginseng is usually well tolerated. Some sources suggest that its use be limited to 3 months because of concerns about the development of side effects.

The most common side effects are headaches and sleep and gastrointestinal problems.

Ginseng can cause allergic reactions.

There have been reports of breast tenderness, menstrual irregularities, and high blood pressure associated with ginseng products, but these products' components were not analyzed, so effects may have been due to another herb or drug in the product.

Ginseng may lower levels of blood sugar; this effect may be seen more in people with diabetes. Therefore, people with diabetes should use extra caution with Asian ginseng, especially if they are using medicines to lower blood sugar or taking other herbs, such as bitter melon and fenugreek, that are also thought to lower blood sugar.

> **Warning!**
> It is important to inform your health care providers about any products containing vitamins, minerals, herbs or other botanicals, amino acids, enzymes, and/or other ingredients intended to supplement the diet. This helps to ensure safe and coordinated care .
> The US Food and Drug Administration has special labelling requirements for dietary supplements and treats them as foods, not drugs.

[www.nccam.nih.gov]

WORD FILE

- **Bark:** corteccia.
- **Burial:** tombale.
- **Burn:** bruciatura.
- **Dietary supplements:** integratori alimentari.
- **Flavor (flavour):** fragranza, profumo.
- **Flaws:** crepe, errori nel disegno sperimentale.
- **Handful:** manciata.
- **Heal (to):** curare, cicatrizzare.
- **Impaired glucose tolerance:** diminuita tolleranza al glucosio.
- **Leaf:** (pl. leaves) foglia.
- **Lung:** polmone.

- **Ointment:** unguento.
- **Root:** radice.
- **Scent:** profumo.
- **Scurvy:** scorbuto.
- **Seed:** seme.
- **Stamina:** resistenza fisica.
- **Stem:** gambo, fusto.
- **Stone carving:** incisione rupestre.
- **Varicose veins:** vene varicose.
- **Wound:** ferita.

Exercise 1

Decide which statements are true (T) or false (F).

		T	F
1.	Bilberry fruit is often used orally as a laxative.	☐	☐
2.	A topical use of aloe includes the treatment of asthma and diabetes.	☐	☐
3.	Aloe was known as the "plant of immortality".	☐	☐
4.	The gel contained by the leaves of aloe is the only part of the plant which is used.	☐	☐
5.	Asian ginseng can have beneficial effects in boosting the immune system.	☐	☐
6.	The leaves of Asian ginseng are dried and then used to make extracts.	☐	☐
7.	Bilberry fruit is commonly used in cooking and tea making.	☐	☐
8.	Deep surgical wounds can receive healing from aloe.	☐	☐
9.	Burns from radiation therapy can be prevented thanks to aloe treatments.	☐	☐
10.	Bilberry fruit is useful in improving night vision.	☐	☐
11.	Exhaustive studies have been carried out on Asian ginseng proving its potential in treating chronic lung infections and Alzheimer's disease.	☐	☐
12.	Ginseng can help in controlling blood pressure.	☐	☐
13.	Patients with diabetes can lower the levels of blood sugar taking ginseng.	☐	☐
14.	There are concerns about possible side effects caused by ginseng which suggest a use limited to 3 months.	☐	☐

Exercise 2

Translate the fragments in italics into English.

1. Aloe vera gel can be found in *centinaia di prodotti per la pelle*, including lotions and sunblocks.

   ....

   ....

2. People with diabetes who use glucose-lowering medication *dovrebbero prestare attenzione* if also taking aloe *per bocca* because preliminary studies suggest aloe may lower blood glucose levels.

   ....

   ....

3. There is not *prove scientifiche sufficienti* to support the use of bilberry fruit or leaf for any health conditions.

4. The root of Asian ginseng contains active chemical components called ginsenosides (or panaxosides) *che si pensa siano* responsible for the herb's medicinal properties.

5. To date, research results on Asian ginseng *non sono sufficientemente decisive* to prove health claims associated with the herb. Only *una manciata* of large clinical trials on Asian ginseng have been conducted.

ECHINACEA

Orally, echinacea is used for treating and preventing the common cold and other upper respiratory infections. Echinacea is also used orally as an immunostimulant for fighting a variety of other infections, including urinary tract infections (UTIs), vaginal candidiasis (yeast infections), genital herpes (HSV Type 1 and 2), nasopharyngeal catarrh, allergic rhinitis, pyorrhea, tonsillitis, streptococcus infections, syphilis, typhoid, malaria, and diphtheria. Other uses include chronic fatigue syndrome (CFS), rheumatism, migraines, dyspepsia, pain, dizziness, rattlesnake bites, swine flu, and attention deficit-hyperactivity disorder (ADHD).
Topically, echinacea is used for boils, abscesses, skin wounds and ulcers, burns, eczema, psoriasis, UV radiation skin damage, herpes simplex, bee stings, and hemorrhoids. Intravenously, echinacea is used for recurrent vaginal candidiasis (yeast infections) and urinary tract infections (UTIs).
Intravenously and intramuscularly, echinacea is used to prolong survival time in patients with advanced hepatocellular carcinoma and colorectal cancer.

Safety

Echinacea is safe when used orally and appropriately, short-term. Several formulations of echinacea have been used safely in trials lasting up to 12 weeks. There is insufficient reliable evidence about the safety of echinacea when used long-term.

Effectiveness

Echinacea is possibly effective in the treatment of common cold. Taking some echinacea preparations seems to modestly reduce symptom severity and duration, possibly by about 10% to 30%. Echinacea seems to be most effective if started when symptoms are first noticed and continued for 7 – 10 days. Not all research is positive as some studies show no benefit for treating the common cold in adults or in children
Taking echinacea orally in combination with a topical antifungal cream seems to be effective for preventing recurrent vaginal yeast infection. Herb juice of Echinacea purpurea in combination with topical econazole lowers recurrence rate to 16.7% compared to 60.5% with econazole alone. Echinacea does not seem effective to prevent or treat recurrent genital herpes infection.

Mechanism of Action

The applicable parts of echinacea are the roots and the above ground parts. The composition of each of the three commonly used echinacea species is similar, with some variation in the amounts of active constituents. Although these species are often used interchangeably, there is very little research comparing them. Echinacea is used for upper respiratory tract infections such as the common cold and influenza infections because it is reported to have antiviral and immune system stimulatory effects; however, there are no reports that it has activity against respiratory viruses.

Echinacea increases phagocytosis and increases lymphocyte activity, possibly by promoting the release of tumor necrosis factor (TNF), interleukin-1 (IL-1), and interferon. Several constituents of echinacea seem to be involved in stimulating this non-specific immune response. Some of these include high-molecular weight polysaccharides, such as heteroxylan and arabinogalactan; and lower molecular weight compounds, including alkylamides and caffeoyl conjugates such as chicoric acid and echinacosides. Heteroxylan might activate phagocytosis, and arabinogalactan seems to induce macrophages to produce the cytokines TNF, IL-1, and interferon beta-2. Macrophages activated by arabinogalactan have been found to be cytotoxic against tumor cells and micro-organisms. The chicoric acid and echinacosides constituents are thought to also play a role in enhancing phagocytosis. Polysaccharides in echinacea also seem to have moderate effects on B-lymphocytes, but no apparent activity on T-lymphocytes. However, echinacea doesn't seem to have any effect on the immune system of healthy volunteers. Some researchers suggest that when echinacea is used for greater than eight weeks, the immunostimulatory effects might decline, making it less effective. To prevent this decline in activity, it is often recommended that a one-week drug holiday be taken after each eight-week treatment period. However, there is no reliable evidence to support either of these claims.

Echinacea's effect on cold symptoms might also result from anti-inflammatory activity. In vitro research suggests constituents of echinacea might inhibit cyclooxygenase and 5-lipoxygenase.

Polyacetylenic compounds in echinacea, including ketoalkenes and ketoalkynes, seem to have antifungal activity, including activity against Candida yeast.

For wound healing, the echinacoside constituent of echinacea seems to protect type III collagen from free radical damage. It also may have activity against bacterial hyaluronidase. Animal research suggests that echinacea extracts can speed would healing, enhance epithelialization, and reduce inflammation. Preliminary information suggests that the caffeoyl constituents of echinacea might help treat or prevent UV radiation skin damage by protecting collagen from free radical damage.

Clinical research using caffeine as a probe for CYP1A2 activity has demonstrated that echinacea can inhibit caffeine clearance by 27%. Echinacea appears to induce hepatic cytochrome P450 3A4 (CYP3A4), but it inhibits intestinal CYP3A4. These opposing effects might result in little or no change in drug levels. More evidence is needed to determine echinacea's affect on drugs metabolized by CYP3A4. Echinacea does not seem to affect cytochrome P450 2C9 (CYP2C9) or 2D6 (CYP2D6) enzymes based on research in humans.

WORD FILE

- **Echinacea:** wild or purple flower commonly found in the US.

- **Bee sting:** puntura d'ape.
- **Clearance:** eliminazione.
- **Enhance (to):** intensificare, aumentare.
- **Wound healing:** cicatrizzante.

Exercise 3

Answer the following questions.

1. Can Echinacea be considered safe in long term treatments?

 ....

 ....

2. Why?

 ....

 ....

3. Can Echinacea be effective in case of common cold?

 ....

 ....

4. Why is it used for the treatment of upper respiratory tracts infections?

 ....

 ....

5. Which is the role of polysaccharides in Echinacea?

 ....

 ....

6. What is the suggestion of researchers for long treatments?

 ....

 ....

7. What are the results of an animal research on this plant?

 ....

 ....

8. What are the effects of caffeoyl constituents in Echinacea?

 ....

 ....

Exercise 4

Complete with the words from the box.

• collagen • activity • research • damage • symptoms • constituents • severity

Echinacea's effect on cold symptoms might also result from anti-inflammatory ....
Taking some echinacea preparations seems to modestly reduce symptom ....
and duration, possibly by about 10% to 30%. Echinacea seems to be most effective if started when .... are first noticed and continued for 7-10 days.
Animal .... suggests that echinacea extracts can speed wound healing, enhance epithelialization, and reduce inflammation. Preliminary information suggests that the caffeoyl .... of echinacea might help treat or prevent UV radiation skin .... by protecting .... from free radicals.

Exercise 5

Decide which statement better fits.

Herbal Medicine, [A] .... referred to [B] .... Herbalism or Botanical Medicine, is the use of herbs for their therapeutic or medicinal value. An herb is a plant or plant part [C] .... for its medicinal, aromatic or savory qualities. Herb plants produce and contain a variety of chemical substances that act [D] .... the body.

Herbal medicine is the [E] .... form of healthcare [F] .... to mankind. Herbs had been [G] .... by all cultures throughout history. It was an integral part of the [H] .... of modern civilization. Primitive man observed and appreciated the great diversity of plants [I] .... to him. The plants [L] .... food, clothing, shelter, and medicine.

[M] .... of the medicinal use of plants seems to have been developed [N] .... observations of wild animals, and by trial and error. As time went on, [O] .... tribe added the medicinal power of herbs in their area to its knowledgebase. They methodically collected information [P] .... herbs and developed well-defined herbal pharmacopoeias. Indeed, well into the 20th century much of the pharmacopoeia of scientific medicine [Q] .... from the herbal lore of native peoples. [R] .... drugs commonly used today are of herbal origin. Indeed, about 25 percent of the prescription drugs dispensed in the United States contain at [S] .... one active ingredient derived from plant material. Some [T] .... from plant extracts; others are synthesized to mimic a natural plant compound.

The World Health Organization (WHO) [U] .... that 4 billion people, 80 percent of the world population, presently use herbal medicine for [V] .... aspect of primary health care. WHO notes that of 119 plant-derived pharmaceutical medicines, [Z] .... 74 percent are used in modern medicine in ways that correlated directly with their traditional uses as plant medicines [X] .... native cultures. Major pharmaceutical companies [Y] .... extensive research on plant materials gathered from the rain forests and other places for their potential medicinal value.

A	1 sometime	2 sometimes	3 times
B	1 as	2 like	3 such
C	1 value	2 valued	3 to value
D	1 of	2 under	3 upon
E	1 older	2 oldest	3 old
F	1 knows	2 known	3 knew
G	1 using	2 use	3 used
H	1 development	2 develop	3 developed
I	1 available	2 challenge	3 increase
L	1 tried	2 provided	3 treated
M	1 many	2 very	3 most
N	1 between	2 within	3 through
O	1 every	2 no	3 each
P	1 on	2 in	3 into
Q	1 is derived	2 was derived	3 has derived
R	1 much	2 very	3 many
S	1 less	2 least	3 at least
T	1 are made	2 were made	3 is made
U	1 provides	2 estimates	3 increases
V	1 any	2 some	3 many
Z	1 on	2 about	3 at
X	1 for	2 by	3 from
Y	1 conducts	2 conduct	3 are conducting

Exercise 6

Fill in the blanks with words from the box.

• originally • worldwide • medications • spread • leaf • blood • relief • more • active • helps • since • broadly • which • breathe

Substances derived from the plants remain the basis for a large proportion of the commercial .... used today for the treatment of heart disease, high .... pressure, pain, asthma, and other problems. For example, ephedra is a herb used in Traditional Chinese Medicine for .... than two thousand years to treat asthma and other respiratory problems. Ephedrine, the .... ingredient in ephedra, is used in the commercial pharmaceutical preparations for the .... of asthma symptoms and other respiratory problems. It .... the patient to .... more easily.

Another example of the use of a herbal preparation in modern medicine is the foxglove plant. This herb had been in use .... 1775. At present, the powdered .... of this plant is known as the cardiac stimulant digitalis to the millions of heart patients it keeps alive ....

Herbal Medicine can be .... classified into various basic systems: Traditional Chinese Herbalism, ... is part of Traditional Oriental Medicine, Ayurvedic Herbalism, which is derived from Ayurveda, and Western Herbalism, which .... came from Greece and Rome to Europe and then .... to North and South America.

COMMON (AND LESS COMMON) MEDICINAL PLANTS

- **Alder buckthorn:** frangula.
- **Autumn crocus:** colchico.
- **Bitter almond:** mandorla amara.
- **Bitter melon:** charante o ampalaya.
- **Black horehound:** ballota.
- **Butcher's broom:** pungitopo.
- **Capsicum:** peperoncino.
- **Carob:** carruba.
- **Cherry Laurel:** lauroceraso.
- **Cinchona:** china.
- **Digitalis:** digitale.
- **English ivy:** edera.
- **Feverfew:** erba amara vera,amarella.
- **Fenugreek:** fieno greco o trigonella.
- **Foxglove:** digitale.
- **German chamomile:** camomilla.
- **Gotu kola:** centella.
- **Hawthorn:** biancospino.
- **Hemlock:** cicuta.
- **Horse chestnut:** ippocastano.
- **Horsetail:** equiseto.
- **Kava kava:** kava.
- **Ipecac:** ipecacuana.
- **Javanese turmeric:** curcuma.
- **Jimson weed:** stramonio.
- **Lavender:** lavanda.
- **Lemon balm:** melissa.
- **Licorice:** liquirizia.
- **Lily-of-the-valley:** convallaria.
- **Mallow:** malva.
- **Marshmallow:** altea.
- **Meadowsweet:** filipendula.
- **Milk thistle:** cardo mariano.
- **Pareira:** curaro.
- **Passion flower:** passiflora.
- **Pheasant's eye:** adonide.
- **Rhatany:** ratania.
- **Rhubarb:** rabarbaro.
- **Senega:** poligala.
- **Siberian ginseng:** eleuterococco.
- **St. John's wort:** erba di S. Giovanni, iperico.
- **Uva Ursi:** uva ursina.
- **Valerian:** valeriana.
- **White horehound:** marrubio.
- **Wormwood:** assenzio.
- **Yarrow:** achillea.

UNIT 14

THE COSMETIC INDUSTRY

A CAREER IN COSMETIC SCIENCE

There are more opportunities today than ever before within the Cosmetic Industry, covering a wide range of disciplines. As the industry becomes more technologically advanced and focused, and the demand grows for products that confer real benefits, rather than just aesthetic appeal, there is an increasing need for scientists to work in both mainstream and specialised areas.

Scientific Research

Research is generally carried out within the larger cosmetic or raw material companies, academic institutions or specialised organisations. There is a growing demand for Pure Research into the properties, behaviour and reaction of skin, hair, teeth and nails at both the macroscopic (Physiological) and microscopic (Biochemical) levels. Some of the actives recently used in cosmetics have been the result of Pharmacological research into topical drugs.

Product Development

There are many companies and specialist consultancies developing ideas for innovative products, as well as the routine products we all use every day such as shampoo, toothpaste, moisturiser, deodorant, etc.

Packaging Development

Besides having instant eye appeal, packaging must be compatible with the product and function safely and effectively in delivering it at the correct rate and in the right amount. Use of the most appropriate material can be critical and all the component parts of the overall pack must fit together and work as a unit. Filling trials need to be carried out to ensure that the pack is practical when subjected to a high speed filling line.

Product Safety and Evaluation

Safety Testing of raw materials may be conducted in vitro, using cell or tissue culture techniques, ex vivo using excised tissue or in vivo, using laboratory animals or (finally) human volunteers. Legislation requires that most new raw materials are tested in laboratory animals, although all animal testing purely for cosmetic purposes has been banned in the UK. There is a continuing trend for in vitro and human volunteer testing protocols to replace animal tests where possible.
Larger companies may have their own safety and evaluation facilities but it is more common to use specialised Contract Research Organisations (CRO), working to international guidelines (GLP –

Good Laboratory Practice or GCP – Good Clinical Practice) and providing an independent assessment of safety or performance.

Microbiology

It is important that microbiologists are involved in the development of a product at an early stage. It needs to be shown that products can withstand reasonable microbial contamination and that the consumer will not be faced with a frightening growth of fungus or bacteria on opening their new product for the first time or after a sustained period of use.

Exercise 1

Answer the following questions.

1. How are tests in cosmetic science carried out?

2. Which are the features of a packaging?

3. How should the involvement of microbiologists be?

COSMETIC SCIENCE

Cosmetic science is a field of study that applies the principles of chemistry and pharmaceutics to the development of cosmetic products, including skin care products and makeup.
Cosmetic scientists conduct applied research to identify new cosmetics ingredients and understand the interactions between various chemical compounds and human skin or hair. Some universities offer master's degrees in cosmetic science; others offer master's degrees in pharmaceutics with a cosmetic science emphasis.

Cosmetic Safety

Safety is the number one priority of the cosmetics industry. There are rigorous regulatory procedures in place to ensure that the cosmetic industry only provides safe products in which consumers can trust.
The safety of cosmetic products is regulated by the European Cosmetics Directive (76/768/EEC), which is implemented in the UK by the Cosmetic Products (Safety) Regulations.
This legislation requires any cosmetic product placed on the market to be safe under normal circumstances of use. A safety assessment must be carried out by the company responsible through a professionally qualified safety assessor for each cosmetic product marketed. This is based on knowledge of the finished product and its ingredients and the assessment is open to inspection by the competent authorities.

In addition, further control is exerted through a list of substances that are prohibited from cosmetics and another list of ingredients that are allowed only when complying with specific restrictions. Where appropriate, there are mandatory warning notices. Certain categories of ingredients (preservatives, UV filters and colorants) may be used only when they have been approved and are listed in the Cosmetics Directive (the so called "positive lists").
In deciding whether or not a substance may be added to the positive lists, the European Commission is advised by a body of independent scientific experts from the member states, the Scientific Committee on Consumer Products (SCCP). The SCCP will study a safety dossier before formulating an opinion, which has to be endorsed by representatives of the member states before a substance can be added to one of the lists of positively approved ingredients.

Exercise 2

Answer the following questions.

1. What does cosmetic science consists of?

2. Which are the requirements for the safety of cosmetics?

3. What does the "positive list" contain?

INGREDIENT LABELING

Like the food industry, the cosmetics industry is subject to mandatory labeling requirements. Product ingredients must be listed on the packaging, on the product itself, or shown in some other way that allows the consumer to be informed. As with food labels, ingredients are listed in descending order by mass or volume. The purpose of this mandatory labeling is to allow consumers to identify ingredients they might be allergic to, and to compare the ingredients in products claiming to have similar benefits.
Products are classified as therapeutic goods rather than cosmetics when they claim to treat an ailment or modify a bodily process. Therapeutic goods are subject to different labeling requirements. Unlike cosmetics, they are required to show only their active ingredients and any ingredients known to have the potential to cause adverse affects in some people. Antiperspirants and anti-dandruff shampoos fall into this category. Cosmetic products are not required to demonstrate their effects scientifically in the same way that therapeutic products are. Their claimed effects are usually couched in cautious language such as 'may reduce the appearance of fine lines and wrinkles'. So consumers should be aware that many of the claims made for cosmetic products have not been scientifically proven.

Exercise 3

Fill in the blanks with words from the box. (Pay attention! They are more than you need.)

• labeling • packaging • scientifically • proven • wrinkles • anti-dandruff • classified • claim • known • adverse effects • trail • allergies

Products are .... as therapeutic goods rather than cosmetics when they .... to treat an ailment or modify a bodily process. Therapeutic goods are subject to different .... requirements. Unlike cosmetics, they are required to show only their active ingredients and any ingredients .... to have the potential to cause .... in some people. Antiperspirants and .... shampoos fall into this category. Cosmetic products are not required to demonstrate their effects .... in the same way that therapeutic products are. Their claimed effects are usually couched in cautious language such as "may reduce the appearance of fine lines and ....". So consumers should be aware that many of the claims made for cosmetic products have not been scientifically .... to be true.

COSMETIC TOXICOLOGY

Unfortunately, sometimes the ingredients in cosmetics can have unintended side-effects. For example, skin allergies (allergic dermatitis) to specific ingredients can be a problem. Allergies to cosmetic products can be due to chemicals such as added fragrances and preservatives. This can lead to a skin rash where the product is applied. If you think you may be allergic to a cosmetic product, it is important to determine which ingredients may be causing the problem. A specialised allergy test, called a patch test, may be helpful in this. Chemicals causing the allergy can then be avoided by reading product labels. Other people, while not allergic to a specific ingredient, may nevertheless find that a product irritates their skin because it damages the outer layers - a condition known as irritant dermatitis.

Exfoliants and skin peels leave the skin underneath temporarily more vulnerable to sun exposure because they remove the outermost protective layer of dead skin cells. Over-washing of hair or skin with soaps and detergents can strip the skin's natural protective oily layer, resulting in dry and scaly skin. Alternatively, excessive use of make-up or oily moisturisers can block pores and aggravate acne. More serious side effects have been suggested for certain cosmetic ingredients. For example, a recent study was published that linked breast cancer with deodorants. The focus of the study was on parabens, a class of chemicals commonly used as preservatives in deodorants and antiperspirants.

While parabens were found in breast cancer tissue, the study did not establish that they were the source of the cancer nor did it identify underarm cosmetics as the source of the chemicals.

A recent US study found that many cosmetics and toiletries used worldwide contained chemicals that were either known cancer-causing agents (carcinogens) or were untested for their effect on human health. More research into the safety of cosmetic chemicals is needed.

In our pursuit of beauty, it is wise to remember that cosmetics can be complex combinations of chemicals. Reading the label and understanding which ingredients are used in a product are helpful when putting on your best face.

Exercise 4

Give the English for the following.

1. Agenti che sono causa di cancro ....
2. Eruzione cutanea ....
3. Effetti collaterali indesiderati ....
4. Strato oleoso ....
5. Lo strato protettivo più esterno ....
6. Idratante oleoso ....
7. Test cutaneo ....
8. Antiforfora ....
9. Conservanti ....

Exercise 5

End sentences in a proper way

1. Side effects to ingredients in cosmetics are sometimes ....
2. A problem for specific ingredients in cosmetics is represented by ....
3. Allergies are often caused by ....
4. Patch tests are useful to determine ....
5. Skin is more vulnerable to sun exposure after the use ....
6. Natural protective oily layer can be ....
7. Accordingly to a recent study there is a link ....
8. Parabens are ....
9. Chemicals contained in cosmetics and toiletries are known as ....
10. People should read the labels to understand ....

WORD FILE

- **Ailment:** disturbo.
- **Anti-dandruff:** antiforfora.
- **Antiperspirant:** antitraspirante.
- **Facilities:** strutture.
- **Layer:** strato.
- **Mainstream:** tradizionale (corrente principale).
- **Mandatory:** obbligatorio, ingiuntivo.
- **Moisturiser:** idratante.
- **Outermost:** il più esterno.
- **Peel (to):** pelare, scorticare.
- **Preservatives:** conservanti.
- **Scaly:** con squame.
- **Toileteries:** articoli d'igiene.
- **Toothpaste:** dentifricio.
- **Underneath:** al di sotto.
- **Wrinkles:** rughe.

COSMETIC GLOSSARY

- **Active ingredient:** the ingredient that is responsible for producing the desired effect of a mixture of ingredients and for giving the product its main characteristic. The active ingredient is not necessarily the most common ingredient in a product.
- **Amino acid:** the basic building block of protein. All amino acids contain an amino (NH2) end, a carboxyl end (COOH) and a side group (R). In proteins, amino acids are joined together when the NH2 group of one forms a bond with the COOH group of the adjacent amino acid.
- **Carcinogen:** a substance that is known to cause cancer.
- **Humectant:** a substance that attracts moisture from the air, retards evaporation and helps hold water.
- **Hydrophilic:** describes a substance that absorbs, dissolves in or is attracted to water.
- **Lead carbonate:** a naturally occurring white amorphous powder with a chemical formula of $PbCO_3$. Used in exterior paints, ceramics, cements, processing of parchment and as a laboratory reagent.
- **Lipophilic:** describes a substance that dissolves in or is attracted to fats, oils or other lipids. Lipophilic functional groups or molecules prefer to be in an environment where there is no water.
- **Occlusion:** the act of closing, shutting or stopping up. In cosmetics this usually refers to a shield or film that is spread onto the skin to slow or prevent moisture evaporation. This shield or film is usually made up of materials, such as oils and waxes that cannot be penetrated by water.
- **Patch test:** test used to identify allergies due to chemicals coming in contact with skin. Individual chemicals are applied separately to the skin and then the skin is observed for reactions over a few days.
- **PH:** the pH scale is used to measure the strength of acids and bases (or alkalis). The acid strength in the human stomach is about pH 2. Alkalis such as caustic soda and basic household cleaners have a pH of about 12 to 14. Neutral is pH 7 (i.e., neither acidic or alkaline).
- **Polymer:** Polymers are large molecules that are made up of many units (monomers) linked together in a chain. There are naturally occurring polymers (e.g., starch and DNA) and synthetic polymers (e.g., nylon and silicone).
- **Polysaccharide:** a carbohydrate made up of a long chain of simple sugar molecules joined together. Starch and cellulose are examples of polysaccharides.
- **Surface tension:** a property of liquid surfaces that causes the surface layer to behave like a thin elastic "skin". Molecules in a liquid have attractive forces that hold them together. Molecules on the surface are attracted to molecules from all sides and below, but not from above.

GRAMMAR FILE

ARTICLES

A/An articolo indeterminativo

An con parole che iniziano per vocale o h muta*
An apple. An hour.

A con parole che iniziano per consonante e suono /ju:/wa/.
A girl. A European country. A car. A garden. A university.

Si usa:

- **con una sola persona o cosa**
  There is a book on the desk.
- **con il rappresentante di un'intera classe**
  A daisy is a flower.
- **con le professioni**
  My sister is a doctor.
- **con le espressioni idiomatiche**
  To have a cold, a headache.
- **con le espressioni numeriche o di misura**
  *Once a week. One hundred kilometres an hour.**
  * h muta: hour, honest, heir, honour.

The articolo determinativo invariabile
Si usa:

- **con nomi di persone o cose già nominati**
  He has a son and a daughter. The son lives in the USA.
- **con alcuni nomi indicanti luoghi** quali *garden, kitchen* (e altre stanze della casa), *cinema, theatre, museum, pub, hotel, restaurant, swimming pool, seaside, country, mountains* etc.
- **con gli aggettivi sostantivati per indicare una categoria di persone o cose**
  The rich and the poor.
- **con i cognomi al plurale** (per indicare tutta la famiglia)
  The Duncans are on holidays.
- **con le lingue ma solo quando accompagnate da "language"**
  English is very important. The English language is getting more and more important.
- **con nomi di fiumi, isole, mari, oceani, catene montuose e nazioni comprendenti le parole State e Kingdom**
  The North Sea. The Thames. The Shetlands. The United States. The United Kingdom.
- **con i nomi di istituzioni**
  The United Nations. The BBC. The CNN. The Bundesbank.

Non si usa mai:

- **con uncountables usati in senso generico**
  Sugar dissolves in water.
- **con sostantivi plurali non specificati** (l'aggettivo qualificativo non specifica)
  Solids have fixed structures. The properties of the matter.
- **con nomi astratti e nomi di colori, religioni e materie**
  Chemistry pertains to the interactions of matter. Blue is my favourite colour. Life can be hard.
- **con i giorni della settimana, mesi, ore**
  Saturday is my favorite day.
- **con i nomi dei pasti e cibi se usati in senso generico**
  Dinner is ready. The dinner Sue cooked for us was fantastic.
- **con le parole: church, university, hospital, school quando usate con riferimento alle attività che vi si svolgono**
  I like school. University is an important step in my life.

Pay attention

So + aggettivo/avverbio (così) *So quick. So stupid. So called.*

So e Such rafforzano il significato.
I was so tired. He was so happy. It was such a nice day. Such nice weather! (Pay attention to the use of the article.) *I thank you so much. He talks so quietly. The book was so good that I couldn't put it down. It was such a good book that I couldn't put it down.*

Such as (come) *Such as sulphuric acid.*

NOUNS

I sostantivi sono di tre generi:

- maschile riferito a persone e animali di sesso maschile: *son, boy, man, king;*
- femminile riferito a persone e animali di sesso femminile; *girl, daughter, woman, queen;*
- neutro riferito a cose o animali in senso generico.

I sostantivi hanno spesso la stessa forma per il femminile e il maschile: *teacher, friend, employee, student.*
Alcuni sostantivi aggiungono il suffisso **ess** per il femminile: *actor/actress, prince/princess.*
Il plurale si forma aggiungendo il suffisso **s** al singolare: *student/students, friend/friends.*

Particolarità:

- i sostantivi che terminano per **s**, **ss**, **sh**, **ch**, **z**, **x** e molti terminanti con **o** prendono il suffisso **es**: *bus/buses, box/boxes, coach/coaches, tomato/tomatoes.* Ma: *radios, pianos, euros;*
- i sostantivi che terminano per **y** preceduta da consonante tramutano la **y** in **i** e poi prendono **es**: *lorry/lorries.* Ma: *boy/boys;*
- alcuni sostantivi che terminano per **f** o **fe** cambiano in **ves**: *wife/wives, leaf/leaves, shelf/shelves, wolf/wolves.* Ma: *roof/roofs, chief/chiefs;*

- alcuni sostantivi hanno plurali completamente diversi: *man/men, woman/women, child/children, mouse/mice, foot/feet, tooth/teeth, ox/oxen, goose/geese*;
- alcuni sostantivi hanno la stessa forma per il singolare e il plurale: *a sheep/two sheep, a fish/three fish, a deer/four deer.*

Pay attention

I cognomi, quando usati a indicare la famiglia, prendono il plurale. *The McDonalds arrived by train.*

COUNTABLE AND UNCOUNTABLE NOUNS

Un **countable noun** può essere preceduto da a/an o da un numero e avere conseguentemente una forma singolare ed una plurale *a boy/two boys, a car/three cars, a man/many men.*
Un **uncountable noun** non può essere preceduto da a/an, né da un numerale e non ha plurale *water, rain, ice, food, money, furniture.*

Pay attention

Alcuni sostantivi numerabili in italiano non lo sono in inglese. Fra questi i più comuni sono:

Advice	➢	consiglio, un consiglio	*A piece of advice*
Information	➢	informazione	*A piece of information; Some information*
Luggage	➢	bagaglio globalmente	*A piece of luggage*
News	➢	notizie	*A piece of news; Some news*
Progress	➢	progresso	*Some progress*
Travel	➢	viaggi	*A trip*
Work	➢	lavoro	*A job*
Money	➢	soldi	*Some money*
Hair	➢	capelli	*Such beautiful hair*
Business	➢	affari	*Business is business*
Homework	➢	compiti	*This is my homework*
Housework	➢	lavori domestici	*She is doing the housework*
Spaghetti	➢		*This spaghetti is delicious!*

Per questo motivo con gli uncountable nouns non si possono usare a/an ma **some**, **any**, **the**, **much (not many)**, **little (not few)**, **such**, **my**, **your** .
Look at the snow outside. I'd like some tea. How much luggage have you got? We've had such wonderful news. They have got much money.

Appartengono al gruppo degli uncountable i nomi di sostanze, malattie, i nomi astratti e quelli che indicano le lingue: *happiness, courage, freedom, salt, butter, flu, water.*
He speaks perfect English e non *He speaks a perfect English.*

Alcuni possono essere countable or uncountable ma con differenze di significato:
A business/businesses ➢ azienda.
A stone/stones ➢ sasso.
A hair/hairs ➢ pelo.
A coffee/two coffees, a tea/two teas, a beer/two beers ➢ due tazze di caffè, due...

ADJECTIVES

Gli aggettivi qualificativi hanno la stessa forma per singolare/plurale, femminile/maschile/neutro.
Janet is English. Tom is English.

L'aggettivo con funzione di attributo, precede sempre il nome a cui si riferisce. È sempre invariabile.
Pandemic measures. Innovative production. Low doses. Previous basic work.

In funzione di predicato segue il verbo **be**.
These studies are famous. The conference hall was empty.

Gli aggettivi dimostrativi hanno una versione singolare e una plurale.
That/those *Those levels. That number.*
This/these *These studies. This vaccine.*
Gli aggettivi di nazionalità hanno sempre l'iniziale maiuscola.

Country	Adjective	People	Noun
Australia	Australian	the Australians	an Australian
Germany	German	the Germans	a German
China	Chinese	the Chinese	a Chinese
Japan	Japanese	the Japanese	a Japanese
England	English	the English	an Englishman
Ireland	Irish	the Irish	an Irishman
Scotland	Scottish*	the Scots	a Scot
Switzerland	Swiss	the Swiss	a Swiss
Wales	Welsh	the Welsh	a Welshman
Denmark	Danish	the Danish	a Dane
Netherland	Dutch	the Dutch	a Dutchman
France	French	the French	a Frenchman
Spain	Spanish	the Spanish	a Spaniard

* *Scotch* riferito a bevande o cibi tipici.

POSSESSIVE ADJECTIVES AND PRONOUNS

Adjectives	Pronouns
My	Mine
Your	Yours
His	His
Her	Hers
Its	Its
Our	Ours
Their	Theirs

Gli aggettivi e pronomi possessivi sono invariabili nel genere e nel numero e non sono mai preceduti dall'articolo.
My friend is British. My friends are American.

Gli aggettivi e pronomi possessivi concordano con il possessore e non con la cosa posseduta:

- **his** quando il possessore è di genere maschile
  ***Tom** and **his** sister are on solida.*
- **her** quando il possessore è di genere femminile
  ***Diana** and **her** brother are at home.*
- **its** quando il possessore è una cosa o un animale
  ***The dog** is black but **its** tail is white.*

Gli aggettivi possessivi sono usati molto più spesso che in italiano e precedono normalmente i nomi delle parti del corpo, vestiario, familiari etc.
He was walking with his hands in his pockets.

L'aggettivo possessivo inglese non è mai preceduto da:

- articolo determinativo;
- articolo indeterminativo;
- aggettivo numerale;
- aggettivo dimostrativo.

In questi casi l'aggettivo possessivo diventa pronome e segue il nome cui si riferisce preceduto da **of**:
Jack is a friend of mine (Jack è un mio amico).
They have got three CDs of mine (Hanno tre miei CD).
I met some friends of his (Ho incontrato alcuni suoi amici).

PRONOUNS

Subjects	Complements
I	Me
You	You
He	Him
She	Her
It	It
We	Us
You	You
They	Them

I pronomi personali soggetto devono essere sempre espressi. I pronomi complemento seguono il verbo o sono accompagnati da preposizioni.
He is working in the lab.
Please come with me!
Can you see him?

TO BE

Affirmative form	Contracted form
I am	I'm
You are	You're
He is	He's
She is	She's
It is	It's
We are	We're
You are	You're
They are	They're

Negative form	Negative contracted form	Interrogative form
I am not	I'm not	Am I?
You are not	You aren't	Are you?
He is not	He isn't	Is he?
She is not	She isn't	Is she?
We are not	We aren't	Are we?
You are not	You aren't	Are you?
They are not	They aren't	Are they?

Il verbo **to be** viene usato:

– come verbo principale e come tale traduce il verbo italiano "essere"
He is my friend. Paris is in France.

– come ausiliare per la forma passiva e i tempi progressivi
This novel was written by Steve H. Ryan. They are watching TV.

– in espressioni idiomatiche quali:
To be old (Avere di anni).
To be cold (Aver freddo).
To be afraid of (Aver paura).
To be right (Aver ragione).
To be hungry (Aver fame).
To be thirsty (Aver sete).
To be wrong (Aver torto).
To be late (Essere in ritardo).
To be hot (Aver caldo).
To be early (Essere in anticipo).

There is – c'è *There is a cat under the table. There is not a cat. Is there a cat?*
There are – ci sono *There are two cars in the parking. There are not the cars. Are there two cars?*

TO HAVE

Affirmative form	Contracted form
I have	I've got
You have	You've got
He has	He's got
She has	She's got
It has	It's got
We have	We've got
You have	You've got
They have	They've got

Negative form	Negative contracted form	Interrogative form
I have not	I haven't	haven't I?

Il verbo **to have** viene usato:

- come **verbo principale** per esprimere possesso (generalmente rafforzato da **got**)
  They have got a nice garden.
- come **verbo ausiliare** per formare i tempi composti
  They have just arrived.
- nelle seguenti espressioni:
  To have breakfast, lunch, dinner – Fare colazione.... *To have a walk* – Fare una passeggiata. *To have a party* – Dare una festa. *To have a coffee/tea* – Prendere.... *To have a bath, shower* – Fare il bagno, doccia.
- per **esprimere un augurio**
  Have a nice day! Have a good time! Have a nice journey!

THE SIMPLE PRESENT

La forma affermativa del **simple present** è data dalla forma base del verbo per tutte le persone tranne che per la terza persona singolare (he/she/it). In questo caso si aggiunge una **s**.
L'infinito è dato dalla **forma base + to: to work** – lavorare.

Affirmative form	I/you/we/they		work
	he/she/it		works
Negative form	I/you/we/they	do not (don't)	work
	he/she/it	does not (doesn't)	work
Interrogative form	Do	I/you/we/they	work
	Does	he/she/it	work
Negative interrogative form	Don't	I/you/we/they	work
	Doesn't	he/she/it	work
Short answers	Yes,	I/you/we/they/he/she/it	do/does
	No,	I/you/we/they/he/she/it	don't/doesn't

Il **simple present** si usa:

- **per indicare azioni abituali**
  I generally catch the 7.15 train. They often go to bed late.
- **per indicare condizioni permanenti** come fatti scientifici o caratteristiche personali e azioni stabilite da orari
  She speaks German. Water boils at 100 °C. The lessons start at 8.30.

Pay attention

3° persona singolare

- verbi che terminano per: **s, ss, sh, ch, z, o, x + es**
  to watch ➢ *he watches* *to bless* ➢ *she blesses*
- verbi che terminano per **y** preceduta da consonante; la y diventa **i + es**
  to try ➢ *he tries* Ma: *to play* ➢ *he plays*

La forma in **ing** corrisponde al gerundio e participio presente italiani.

Forma base + ing

go/going, read/reading.

Si usa:

- **dopo le preposizioni**: *before writing, without using, after reading.*
- **dopo alcuni verbi come mind, avoid, hate, enjoy, like, love**
  Do you mind closing the door? I like cycling. She hates taking drugs.
- **nelle forme progressive**
  Those patients are taking paracetamol tablets. The doctor is writing a prescription.

Pay attention

Take ➢	*taking*	"e" muta finale cade.
Stop ➢	*stopping*	raddoppio consonante finale nei monosillabici.
Prefer ➢	*preferring*	raddoppio consonante finale nei bisillabici quando preceduta da una vocale accentata.
Lie ➢	*lying*	"ie" dittongo finale diventa "y". Ma: *study/studying, play/playing.*

THE IMPERATIVE

L'imperativo affermativo è dato dalla forma base del verbo, cioè dall'infinito senza il "to".
State the dose. Give instructions. Sign the prescription.

La prima persona plurale è formata da **let + complemento + forma base verbo**.
Let us (let's) read this article. Let's go!

Imperativo negativo: **don't + forma base verbo**.
Don't write a prescription. Don't call the doctor.

Nella lingua scritta il divieto è spesso reso da **no + ing form**.
No smoking. No parking.

THE PRESENT CONTINUOUS

È formato dal verbo **to be (declinato) + la forma in "ing" del verbo base**.
They are studying. He is working.

Poiché è presente il verbo "to be" le forme interrogative e negative seguono lo schema di questo verbo.
The child isn't playing. Is the child playing? Yes, he is/No, he isn't.

È usato per:

- **indicare un'azione in corso di svolgimento**. In questo caso è spesso accompagnato da *now*, *at the moment*, *today*, *at present* etc.
  The child is playing in the garden – Ora, in questo momento sta giocando.
- **indicare un'azione futura già programmata o stabilita**. In questo caso è spesso accompagnato da espressioni di tempo quali *soon, tomorrow, next month, in two hours* etc.
  They are going to the cinema tonight – Non è ancora sera, indica quindi un'azione futura.

Il simple present e il present continuous non hanno la stessa funzione. Il primo indica uno stato di cose o un'azione abituale.
It often snows in winter.

Il secondo un'azione in corso in un determinato momento del presente.
Don't get out. It's snowing.

Pay attention

Alcuni verbi sono usati quasi sempre nella forma del simple present. Sono i verbi che si riferiscono a:

- **mental states**: understand, believe, know, imagine, forget, think, remember, suppose, realise, recognize etc.;
- **likes and dislikes**: hate, like, love, wish, dislike etc.

THE SIMPLE FUTURE

Il **futuro semplice** si forma premettendo gli ausiliari **shall** e **will** alla forma base del verbo.
Shall viene di norma usato per la prima persona singolare e plurale ma nell'inglese informale si preferisce will per tutte le persone.
Shall e *will* sono quasi sempre usati nella forma contratta che è *'ll* per entrambi.

Affirmative form	I/you/he, she, it/we/you/they	will ('ll)	work
Negative form	I/you/he, she, it/we/you/they	will not won't	work
Interrogative form	will	you/he, she, it/we/you/they	work?
Negative interr. form	won't	you/he, she, it/we/you/they	work?
Short answers	Yes, No,	you/he, she, it/we/you/they	will won't

Il simple future è usato:

- **per prevedere eventi futuri** che non dipendono dal volere di chi parla
  The course will start next week. The lecturer won't meet the students.
- **per indicare la disponibilità** o fare una **promessa**
  I'll take you to the chemist's. They'll lend us their books.

- **con i verbi hope, think, be sure, believe, suppose**, in italiano seguiti da infinito
  I'm sure he'll get a scholarship. He hopes he'll take part in the meeting.
- **nelle frasi principali collegate a proposizioni condizionali o temporali**
  You'll feel better if you take this tablet.
- **per indicare un'azione che si decide di compiere all'istante**
  It's late. I'll take a taxi.

In italiano capita di avere frasi principali al futuro con subordinate introdotte da *quando, se, non appena, finché* anch'esse al futuro. In inglese solo la principale è al futuro e la frase introdotta da *when, if, as soon as, as long as* è al presente.
You'll follow this treatment as long as you don't feel better. When you feel better you'll stop taking these drugs.

TO BE GOING TO

To be going to è usato per esprimere:

- **l'intenzione a compiere un'azione**
  I am going to buy a new car.
- **un evento imminente ritenuto certo o inevitabile**
  It's cloudy. It's going to rain.

Pay attention

Poiché in questa forma è presente il verbo "to be" le forme negative, interrogative, interrogativo-negative e le risposte seguono lo schema del verbo "to be".
Is it going to rain? No, it isn't.

THE SIMPLE PAST

Verbi regolari: forma base + ed, unica forma per tutte le persone.
to work/worked.

Verbi irregolari: vedi dizionari dove appaiono nella sequenza presente, passato, participio passato
to go/went/gone.
Il verbo **to be** ha una passato particolare:
to be, was/were, been è il paradigma.
Simple past: *I was, you were, he/she/it was, we were, you were, they were.*

Negative form	**soggetto + did + not + forma base del verbo** (did not – didn't) *They worked. They did not work.*
Interrogative form	**did + soggetto + forma base del verbo** *They watched TV. Did they watch TV?*
Short answers	**yes + soggetto + did** **no + soggetto + did not** *Did you go to the cinema? Yes, I did* *No, I didn't.*

Pay attention

Quando il verbo termina per "e" si aggiunge solo "d": *to live* ➣ *he lived.*
Quando è monosillabico terminante con una sola consonante preceduta da vocale raddoppia la consonante: *to stop* ➣ *she stopped.*
Quando è bisillabico preceduto da vocale accentata raddoppia la consonante finale: *to travel* ➣ *we travelled.*
Quando termina per "y" preceduta da consonante tramuta la "y" in "i" prima di "ed": *to study* ➣ *they studied, to play* ➣ *they played.*

Il **Simple Past** si riferisce sempre ad azioni completamente trascorse. È spesso accompagnato da espressioni di tempo determinato quali *yesterday*, *last week*, *two years ago*, *last night* etc.
I went to the USA two years ago. I didn't go to school yesterday. I broke my leg skiing last month.

Quando però l'azione non è ancora completamente conclusa, o pur riguardando il passato ha ancora attinenza con il presente, si usa il **Present Perfect**.
Present Perfect: **has/have + past participle**.
I study English. I studied English last year. I have studied English.

Il **Present Perfect** è spesso accompagnato da: *just* (appena), *already* (già), *not ... yet* (non ancora), *recently*, *never*, *many times*, *all day* etc.
Forma negativa, interrogativa e short answers come con il verbo to have.

Simple Past	**Present Perfect**
I went to the USA two years ago	*I haven't been to the USA yet*
I didn't go to school yesterday	*I haven't been to school today*
I broke my leg skiing last month	*I have just broken my leg*

CONDITIONAL

Il condizionale presente si forma con gli ausiliari: **should** e **would + verbo base**. *Should* è per la prima persona singolare e plurale. Nelle frasi affermative should e would vengono contratti in **'d**.

Affirmative form	*I'd be glad to come to your party.*
Negative form	*I wouldn't marry him.*
Interrogative form	*Would you marry him?*

Il condizionale presente viene usato per esprimere un'ipotesi, un'eventualità.
In case of fire, what would you do?
Il condizionale del verbo *to like* ha una valenza particolare (v. p. 139).

IF CLAUSE

Si riferisce ad azioni che possono verificarsi ma con scarsa probabilità.

Main clause:	**if clause*:**
condizionale presente	if + passato semplice
I would buy you a present...	*... if I had enough money*

* Con il verbo essere è spesso usato were per tutte le persone. Soprattutto in situazioni fortemente ipotetiche.
If I were the President of the USA I would stop the war.

DURATION FORM

È usata per esprimere azioni o situazioni che sono iniziate nel passato ma che sono ancora in corso.
La duration form è resa con il **present perfect** o con il **present perfect continuous**

Present perfect	con i **verbi che non vogliono la forma progressiva** come i verbi di stato sentimento, percezione etc. *I have been here in New York since 2004.* **Nelle frasi negative**: *I haven't seen him for two years.*
Present perfect continuous	con i **verbi che permettono l'uso della forma ing** *I have been waiting for him since 4 o'clock.*

FOR/SINCE

Traducono la preposizione italiana "da".

For: quantità di tempo.
How long? *How long have you been studying chemistry? For three years.*

Since: momento preciso in cui ha inizio un'azione.
Since when? *Since when have you been studying chemistry? Since the beginning of this school year.*

THE PASSIVE FORM

La forma passiva è data dal verbo **to be (nel tempo adeguato) + past participle** del verbo indicante l'azione.

Present simple	*Those computers are made in Japan.*
Present continuous	*Dinner is being cooked now.*
Past simple	*Smoking was not allowed.*
Past continuous	*Dinner was being cooked when I arrived.*
Present perfect	*Those letters have been written by Tom.*
Past perfect	*The fire had already been lit.*
Future	*The patient is going to be visited; The patient will be dismissed at the end of the week.*

Il progressivo passivo **is-are/was-were + being** sottolinea l'azione in corso.
A school is being built. A new lab is being equipped.

Il complemento d'agente è spesso sottinteso. Quando indicato è espresso da **by**.
This drug is well tolerated. The house is being renovated. My car is being washed. Those computers were imported by his company.

Nella lingua inglese si fa ricorso alla forma passiva molto più che in italiano.
In particolare la forma passiva viene usata:

- quando si vuole sottolineare l'azione e non chi l'ha compiuta; spesso in questo caso il complemento d'agente è omesso
  A mechanic is repairing my car – stress su *mechanic*.

My car is being repaired – stress sull'azione di *repairing*.
Paracetamol was introduced into clinical practice in 1893. Attenzione = hanno introdotto il paracetamolo.

- quando non si sa di preciso chi ha compiuto una determinata azione
  Students were requested not to smoke.
- nel linguaggio tecnico e scientifico, soprattutto per illustrare procedimenti e descrivere procedure
  The table is based on analgesic drugs.
- negli avvisi, nelle istruzioni, negli articoli di giornali
  Topical use is not recommended.
- quando si scrive in modo formale (relazioni, reports, lettere etc)
  It was agreed to accept her proposal. It was considered to be an acceptable alternative.
- nel riportare informazioni
  The minister is said to be in favour of.... He is considered to be the most famous scientist in the field of.... This is thought to be the most important invention of this century.

Le varie forme impersonali usate in italiano quali, ad esempio, si dice, si pensa, si ritiene, la gente dice, pensano, credono etc. vengono rese in inglese con il passivo.
Topical antihistamines are considered useful for the relief of allergic conjunctivitis. We were said that this dosage is rarely required. The patients are required to wait in this room.

MODAL VERBS

I verbi modali sono di norma usati con altri verbi per esprimere, possibilità, obbligo, permesso, probabilità, volontà etc.

- **Hanno una sola forma per tutte le persone.**
- **Sono sempre seguiti dalla forma base del verbo.**
- **Non richiedono l'uso del to do nella forma negativa, interrogativa o negativo-interrogativa.**

Can May – potere

Per esprimere **la capacità di fare qualcosa** si usa:

– **can**	per indicare ciò che si sa o non si sa fare al **presente** *I can use a computer. They can speak German.*
– **could**	per indicare ciò che si sapeva o non si sapeva fare al **passato** *I could ski very well when I was a child. He could not leave last week. He was ill in bed.*

Per **chiedere, concedere o rifiutare un permesso**:

– **can**	per chiedere un permesso *Can I use your computer?*
– **could/may/might**	per chiedere un permesso in modo formale *Could you call me back, please? May we park in your garden? Might they leave the lecture?*
– **can**	per concedere o rifiutare un permesso *Can I take your car? No, you can't. Can I park here? Yes, you can./No, you can't. You can take the oral exam because you have passed the written one.*

Per **esprimere richieste**:

– **can**	informale *Can you pass me that book?*
– **could**	più formale e cortese *Could you show me your badge, please?*

Per indicare **la probabilità**:

– **may/might**	might esprime maggiore incertezza *The computer store may be closed on Saturday afternoon.* *Dr Sullivan might be in the library.*
– **to be able to**	verbo sostitutivo seguito dalla forma base del verbo sostituisce **can** e **could** nei tempi che non sono simple present, simple past e present conditional *He will be able to use the computer at the end of this computering session.* *I haven't been able to see your report yet.*
– **to be likely to**	verbo sostitutivo di **may** e **might** con il significato di probabilità *They'll be likely to come.*
– **to be allowed to/ to be permitted to**	verbi sostitutivi con il significato di avere il permesso *Next year, students will be allowed to use this lab.*

Quando "potere" al passato non si riferisce tanto a una capacità o abilità ma piuttosto a una situazione occasionale si preferisce usare **to manage** o **to be able to**.
He could play the piano when he was 8. We managed to make some progress after hours of negotiation.

Pay attention

Could e **might** corrispondono anche al condizionale.
I could try to call him at home. I might be too late for him.

How to Translate "volere"

Will presente "volere".
Seguito dalla forma base del verbo e usato anche per costruire il futuro

- **esprime una richiesta formale**
  Will you wait here?
- **una decisione istantanea**
  This is a good idea. I'll follow it.
- **una promessa**
  Will you help me?

Would like il condizionale di "like" traduce il nostro "volere" nei seguenti casi:

- **offrire qualcosa**
  Would you like a cup of coffee? Would you like any help?
- **fare inviti**
  Would you like to take part to the meeting?

- **esprimere un desiderio o una richiesta**
  I would like to be rich. I would like some beer, please

Il verbo italiano **volere che + congiuntivo** viene reso con:
to want + complemento oggetto + infinito
Mary wants me to help her. Do you want me to go home?

Questa costruzione è usata anche con **would like, would prefer, would expect**.
They did not want the students to enter the library. Dad would prefer you to stay at home tonight. I would like my daughter to go abroad this summer.

La forma italiana "volerci" seguita da complemento di tempo si traduce con il verbo **to take**.
It takes ten minutes to go to the airport. I took ten minutes to go to the airport. How long does it take to go back?

Would rather + infinito: preferire
I would rather go to the cinema. I'd rather go back immediately. I'd rather not go out tonight. I'm tired.

Must – dovere (tempo presente)

Viene usato per indicare:
- **obbligo**
  Investigators must try both methods to make the comparison useful.
- **deduzione**
  This drug is useful in case of hayfever. It must be an antihistaminic. He must be American.
- **consiglio**
  You must take into consideration the placebo effects.

Il verbo **to have to** sostituisce "must" nei tempi mancanti e viene, comunque, utilizzato per esprimere:
- **obbligo o necessità derivante da condizioni o circostanze**
  We did not get any results. We have to carry out a new test. I have to drive to work every day.
- **un non obbligo**
  You don't have to wait for me.

Shall

Corrisponde alle prima persona singolare e plurale interrogative del presente del verbo "dovere". Si usa per:
- **offrire aiuto** chiedendo il parere o la volontà altrui (devo? Vuoi/volete che io...? Volete che noi...?)
  Shall I open the window? Shall we carry out the test for you?
- **fare una proposta**
  Shall we start working? Shall we call our tutor?

Should

È il condizionale del verbo "dovere". Può esprimere:
- **consiglio, suggerimento**
  You should check your results. They should collect more data.

- **dovere, obbligo**
  You should study harder.
- **rimprovero**
  You should pay attention to the laboratory results.

Ought to

È sinonimo di should.

Pay attention

Must e **have to** sono spesso intercambiabili.

Must	Have to
We use **must** when the speaker feels that something is necessary - *You **must** exercise (I'm telling you).* - *You **must** be quiet (I'm telling you).* **Must** can also express a wish - *I **must** buy a newspaper. I want to see the football results.* - *We **must** invite Jenny. She is so lovely.*	We use **have to** when the situation make something necessary - *I **have to** exercise (the doctor told me).* - *We **have to** be quiet (that's the rule).* - *I **have to** buy a newspaper. The boss asked me to get one.* - *We **have to** invite Tom and Debby. They invited us last time.*
Mustn't	**Needn't**
We use **mustn't** to say that something is a bad idea - *You **mustn't** drop your glasses. They'll break.* - *You **mustn't** forget your keys or you won't get in.*	We use **needn't** when something is not necessary - *You **needn't** wash your car. It's clean.* - *We **needn't** make sandwiches. There is a small restaurant in the village.*

DATES

Gli anni si leggono come segue:

1985 nineteen eighty five.
1999 nineteen ninty nine.
1900 nineteen hundred.
2003 two thousand and three.
2010 two thousand and ten.

La data può essere espressa come segue:
14 March, March 14, 14th March, March 14th, 14/3/2007 (UK), 3/14/2007 (USA).

Months: January, February, March, April, May, June, July, August, September, October, November, December.

Days: Sunday, Monday, Tuesday, Wednesday, Thursday, Friday, Saturday.

On	In	At
14 March	March	the beginning of March
Monday	summer	the weekend
Wednesday morning	2007	Christmas
my birthday	the morning/the afternoon/the evening	night
		six o'clock

COMPOUND NOUNS

Sono composti da due o più sostantivi. Solo l'ultimo nome mantiene il proprio valore di sostantivo. Gli altri assumono la valenza di aggettivi e in quanto tali sono invariabili: *influenza virus*, *chicken eggs*, *vaccine production process*.
Il primo sostantivo, di solito, risponde alla domanda e.g. *What kind?*: *car factory*, *city centre*, *work experience*, *kitchen table* etc.
Ma nonostante quanto detto sopra *accounts department*, *savings account*, *sports car*, *clothes store* etc.

COMPARATIVES

– Aggettivi/avverbi:	**as... as**	in frasi affermative *Lucy is as tall as Mary.*
	not so/as... as	in frasi negative *My bike is not so new as yours. My bike is not as new as yours.*
– Sostantivi:	**as much... as**	con sostantivi singolari *I've got as much money as you.*
	as many... as	con sostantivi plurali *I bought as many books as you.*

Quando il secondo termine di paragone è espresso da un pronome personale, questo è reso con un pronome soggetto, se è seguito da un ausiliare. Altrimenti si preferisce il pronome complemento (meno formale).

Il **comparativo e superlativo di maggioranza** degli aggettivi si formano:
- aggiungendo i suffissi **er/est** (con the davanti) in caso di aggettivi monosillabici o bisillabici terminanti in y, er, le, ow.

Nice	nicer	the nicest
Happy	happier	the happiest
Cold	colder	the coldest
Clever	cleverer	the cleverest
Narrow	narrower	the narrowest

- Facendo precedere gli aggettivi da **more** o **the most**.

Interesting	more interesting	the most interesting
Boring	more boring	the most boring

Il secondo termine di paragone dei comparativi è introdotto da **than**.
Mr Greenwood is older ***than*** *Mr Smith. This kind of drugs are more effective* ***than*** *paracetamol.*

Il secondo termine di paragone nei superlativi di maggioranza è introdotto da:
- **in** se riferito a un luogo e con espressioni quali: in my class, in my team, in my family
  He is the most experienced manager in this company. This is the most recent building in our town.
- **of** con le espressioni di tempo e con i plurali riferiti a un gruppo
  It was the best week of the year. Larry is the oldest of my brothers.

Pay attention

Prima di aggiungere i suffissi "er" o "est" occorre tener conto delle seguenti regole ortografiche:
- se l'aggettivo termina con una sola consonante preceduta da un'unica vocale, la consonante finale raddoppia: hot/hotter/the hottest.
- la "e" finale viene omessa: fine/finer/the finest.
- la "y" preceduta da consonante si trasforma in "i": lucky/luckier/the luckiest.

Adjectives	Irregular comparatives	Irregular superlatives
Good/well	better	the best
Bad/badly	worse	the worst
Far	farther (+ lontano) further (ulteriore)	the farthest the furthest
Much/many	more	the most
Little	less	the least
Late	later	the last (ultimo in senso assoluto) the latest (il più recente)
Near	nearer	the next (prossimo, successivo) the nearest (il più vicino)
Old	older elder	the oldest the eldest*

* Usato solo per persone (anziano) soprattutto familiari e mai nelle comparazioni.

Il **comparativo di maggioranza** con i **sostantivi e gli avverbi** si forma con **more**.
They have got more money than me. I have passed more exams than you. We did it more easily than we thought.

Il comparativo può essere rafforzato da **much/a lot** o minimizzato da **a bit/slightly**.
How do you feel? Much better – Come ti senti? Molto meglio.
Do not go by train. It's a lot more expensive – Non prendere il treno. È molto più costoso.

Diversamente dall'italiano il **superlativo relativo** riferito a due cose o persone si rende con il comparativo preceduto dall'articolo "the".
Which is the more interesting of these two books? – Qual è il più interessante di questi due libri?
This is the more effective of the two tests – Questo è il più efficace dei due test.

Attenzione alle seguenti espressioni italiane che sono così rese:
- Il suo inglese sta diventando sempre migliore – *His English is getting* ***better and better***.
- Sempre più gente arriva per il concerto – ***More and more*** *people are arriving for the concert.*
- Più piccola è l'auto, più facile è parcheggiarla – ***The smaller*** *the car,* ***the easier*** *it's the parking.*
- Prima arrivano e meglio è – ***The sooner*** *they arrive,* ***the better***.

Il **comparativo e il superlativo di minoranza** si formano premettendo rispettivamente **less** e **the least**.
The new treatment is less painful than the old one – La nuova cura è meno dolorosa di quella vecchia.
This is the least interesting book I've ever read – Questo è il libro meno interessante che abbia mai letto.

Il secondo termine di paragone si esprime come nel comparativo di maggioranza.
Diovan is less effective than Tekturna. Tom is the least boring of my friends. Jane is the least experienced analyst in this company.

Il comparativo di minoranza con i sostantivi si forma premettendo **less** ai sostantivi singolari e **fewer** a quelli plurali.
He came to see me less often than I hoped. I have less money than my brother. There are fewer students than in the past.

ENOUGH (ABBASTANZA)

È posto dopo aggettivi ed avverbi e prima dei sostantivi.
I can't run fast. I'm not fit enough. Is Joe experienced enough for the job?/Does he have enough experience? It is high enough. I haven't got enough energy. We have enough money.

PARTITIVES

Some viene usato in:

– **frasi affermative**	*I've got some new books. There is some coffee for you*
– **frasi interrogative**	quando si esprimono offerte o richieste *Would you like some coffee? Can I have some water, please?*

Any viene usato in:

– **frasi interrogative**	*Are there any letters for me?*
– **frasi negative**	*There aren't any books on the desk*
– **frasi dubitative**	*I don't know if there are any students in the library*

No corrisponde a nessuno, niente. Può sostituire l'espressione **not... any***.
I haven't got any time/I've got no time. There weren't any students/There were no students. No student can carry out this job.

* In inglese non si possono avere due negazioni nella stessa frase.

Pay attention
Any si usa anche in frasi affermative ma con il significato di qualunque, qualsiasi.
Call me any time. Give me any pen.

INDEFINITE PRONOUNS

	Affirmative	Interrogative		Negative	
	Some	**Any**	**Any**	**No**	**Every**
People	somebody anyone *qualcuno*	anybody not... anyone *qualcuno*	not... anybody no one *nessuno*	nobody everyone *nessuno*	everybody *tutti/ognuno*
Things	something *qualcosa*	anything *qualcosa*	not... anything *niente/nulla*	nothing *niente/nulla*	everything *tutto/ogni cosa*
Places	somewhere *da qualche parte*	anywhere *da qualche parte*	not... anywhere *da nessuna parte*	nowhere *da nessuna parte*	everywhere *da ogni parte/ dappertutto*

I composti di some e body hanno lo stesso valore. Sono usati solo per le persone e il verbo è sempre al singolare.
Someone wants to speak to you. Somebody is waiting for Dr Lewis.
Everybody was happy for him – Erano tutti felici per lui.

Avverbi e pronomi indefiniti seguono le stesse regole di some, any e no.
There was nothing we could do for him. Can you see my keys anywhere? I went nowhere. Nobody asked to see him. I didn't meet anybody at his party. Did you meet anybody at my party? I met someone at her party.

Contrariamente all'italiano non richiedono alcuna preposizione.
Qualcosa di interessante – *Something interesting.*
Qualcosa di nuovo – *Something new.*

All'inizio delle frasi negative e nelle risposte brevi si usano: nobody, no one, nothing e nowhere.
Nobody is attending Dr Rice's lecture. What were they doing? Nothing.

INTERROGATIVE PRONOUNS AND ADJECTIVES

Who	Chi? (soggetto*)	*Who is your tutor?*
Who(m)	Chi? (complemento)	*Who did you meet at the party?* *Who are you waiting for?*
What	Che cosa? Quale? (pronome/aggettivo; soggetto/complemento)	*What's your favourite colour?* *What colour is your car?*
Which	Quale? (pronome/aggettivo)	*Which football team do you like?* *Which of these sports is your favourite one?*
Whose	Di chi?	*Whose book is this?* *Whose is this book?*
How	Come? In che modo?	*How tall are you?* *How can I get to the station?*
How many	Quanti?	*How many tickets have you got?*
How many times	Quante volte?	*How many times have you visited the US?*

* I pronomi interrogativi soggetto non vogliono l'inversione del verbo e l'uso degli ausiliari.

How long	Quanto tempo? Da quanto tempo? Per quanto tempo?	*How long does it take to get to the airport?* *How long have you been living here?* *How long are you going to stay here?*
What about? + ing form	Che...?	*What about going to the cinema?* *What about Debbie?*
Why*	Perché?	*Why are they so late? Sorry, I don't know why.*

* Nelle interrogative dirette e indirette, *because* nelle risposte.

What: che, che cosa, quale? Usato anche quando si vuole conoscere il tipo o il genere di qualcosa o a fronte di una larga scelta.
What size in this shirt?

Which: che, che cosa, quale? Usato solo in riferimento a una scelta tra un numero limitato di cose o persone.
What factors cause this disease? Here are the drugs. Which drug did he take?

Quando il pronome interrogativo è usato con una preposizione questa viene posta alla fine della frase.
Where does the patient come from? What's this abstract about?

	Persons	**Things or animals**
Subject	who/that	which/that
Complement	whom/that	which/that
With prepositions	preposizione + whom	preposizione + which

RELATIVE PRONOUNS

I pronomi relativi sono invariabili per genere e numero. Le frasi relative possono essere :
- **defining** o **non incidentali** quando sono indispensabili all'identificazione di una cosa o di una persona. Queste frasi non sono mai precedute da virgola;
- **non-defining** o **incidentali** quando forniscono indicazioni suppletive, non essenziali all'identificazione di una cosa o una persona. Questo tipo di frasi è sempre racchiuso fra due virgole.

Relative Pronouns: subjects

Nelle frasi **non incidentali** i pronomi soggetto sono **who** o **that** per le persone, **which** o **that** per cose o animali.
The girl who/that is speaking to Joe is my daughter. The car which/that is over there is mine. Dr Grant is the surgeon who/that carried out the operation. The tests which/that were carried out in the US proved this drug potential.

I pronomi relativi soggetto non possono mai essere omessi. Possono invece essere omessi quando hanno la funzione di complemento specialmente nel linguaggio informale.
Have you read the report (which/that) Dr Foreman wrote?

Nelle frasi **incidentali** i pronomi soggetto sono **who** per le persone e **which** per le cose e gli animali. **That** non viene mai usato.
My friend Brian, who is a doctor, lives in the US; Professor Coleman, who is a specialist in this field, will speak to the audience.

Relative Pronouns: objects

Nelle frasi **non incidentali** si usa **who/that** per le persone e **which/that** per le cose ed animali. Nel linguaggio formale sono spesso omessi.
The girl (who/that) you met at the lecture is a new student.

Nelle frasi **incidentali** sono **who(m)** e **which**. That non è mai usato. Questi pronomi non possono essere omessi.
Mr White, who(m) you met in New York, is now living in Paris.

Quando un pronome relativo è usato con una preposizione di norma viene omesso e la preposizione viene posta in fondo alla frase relativa.
I've just seen the report (which) you were talking about yesterday. The lady I was speaking to is our new teacher.

Il relativo **whose** indica il possesso e traduce l'italiano "il cui/la cui/i cui/le cui". È invariabile e non viene mai omesso. È immediatamente seguito dal nome della persona o cosa posseduta.
Dr Duncan whose article on paracetamol has aroused a lot of controversy, will take part to the conference.
The researcher whose curriculum you read yesterday is waiting for you in the library.

Where traduce le espressioni in cui/dove.
The library where I spend my afternoons is very quiet. The York Hospital, where Sue works, is looking for staff.

Which può essere usato in riferimento a un'intera frase. Traducendo "il che/la qual cosa".
I gave all my exams in June, which wasn't easy.

What ciò che/quello che.
I understand what you mean. We saw what they did.

All (that) tutto ciò che.
This is all I have got.

HOW TO TRANSLATE "MOLTO, MOLTI"

Sostantivo singolare	**much/a lot of**:
– frase affermativa	*There is a lot of coffee/much coffee.*
– frase negativa	*There isn't much coffee.*
– frase interrogativa	*Is there much coffee?*
Sostantivo plurale	**many/a lot of/lots of**:
– frase affermativa	*There are a lot of cars /lots of cars. There are many cars.*
– frase negativa	*There aren't many cars.*
– frase interrogativa	*Are there many cars?*
Forme verbali	**a lot/much/very much**
nelle frasi affermative si preferisce "a lot"	*He always reads a lot.*
	Sue doesn't read much.
Aggettivo o avverbio very	*It's very late. They arrived very quickly.*

Fairly/rather/quite + adjectives and adverbs:
- fairly: abbastanza/positive meaning *Fairly well*
- rather: abbastanza;
- quite: abbastanza/completamente.

Pay attention

In American English very è spesso "quite".
That dress is quite nice/That dress is very nice.

Quite ha il significato di "completely" in British English.

BOTH, EITHER, NEITHER

Both, **either** e **neither**: sono usati per due cose o persone. Possono essere usati da soli (non accompagnati da pronomi o nomi).
The store has two lifts and both are out of order. Neither is working.

Both: the one and the other.
Tom and Joe are both students. I met them both in the library.

Either: the one or the other.
I have met either twin/either of the twins/either of them.

Neither: not the one or the other.
Neither shoe fits/neither of the shoes fit(s)/neither of them fit(s).

PREPOSITIONS OF PLACE

Prepositions of Place

Above	su, sopra (senza contatto) *There is a lamp above the door.*
On	su, sopra (con contatto) *The cat is on the chair. The picture is on the wall.*
Over	sopra *The sky is over us. The plane is over the sea*
Among	tra (più di due) *There is a child among us.*
Between	tra (due cose o persone) *Sue is sitting between Joe and Mary.*
Below	sotto *Below sea level.*
Under	sotto *They found the cat under a bridge.*
Behind	dietro *There is a tree behind the house. The bank is behind the library.*
In	in, a, dentro *Sue is in Milan, in Oxford Street, in the kitchen.*
At	a *Sue is at the restaurant, at school, at the bus stop, at 20 Cannon Street, at a party, at a lecture.*

In front of	davanti a (generico) *The children were sitting in front of the TV set.*
Opposite	dirimpetto, di fronte a *The bank is opposite the library.*
Inside	dentro *The dog is inside the garden.*
Outside	fuori *He is standing outside the door.*
Near	vicino a *The chair is near the window. Monza is near Milan.*
Close to	vicino a *Close to the park.*
Next to	accanto a *There is a baker's next to the library.*
In the middle of	nel mezzo di *There is a fountain in the middle of the park.*

Prepositions of Movement

Across	attraverso, per *He run across the road.*
Along	lungo *Go along Melville Road and then…*
Down	giù *They walked down Bond Street.*
From	da *They'll arrive from Paris.*
Into	in *I went into the shop.*
Out of	fuori di *Take the keys out of your bag.*
Past	dopo, oltre *Go past the station and turn into Channel Street.*
Through	attraverso, per *Go through the main entrance.*
To	a, in, da *I went to London.*
Up	su *The dog ran up a tree.*

Pay attention

To be at home	➢	essere a casa	*We spent the evening at home*
To go home	➢	andare a casa	*Are you going home?*

VERBS + PREPOSITIONS/ADVERBS

Up	
To get up	alzarsi
To give up	rinunciare
To grow up	crescere/coltivare
To ring up	telefonare
To stand up	alzarsi (in piedi)
To wake up	svegliarsi
Out	
To carry out	condurre, svolgere, realizzare
To find out	trovare/scoprire
To go out	uscire
To put out	spegnere (fuoco/sigaretta)
On	
To carry on	continuare, proseguire, svolgere
To get on	salire (mezzo di trasporto)
To go on	continuare
To keep on	continuare
To put on	indossare
To switch on	accendere (luce, gas, etc.)
To turn on	accendere, aprire (rubinetto)
In	
To come in	entrare
To fill in	compilare (modulo), riempire
Off	
To get off	scendere (mezzo di trasporto)
To put off	rimandare,postporre
To set off	mettere in moto, ripartire
To switch off	spegnere (luce, gas, etc.)
To turn off	spegnere (luce, gas, etc.) + rubinetto
To take off	togliersi (indumenti), decollare
After	
To look after	badare/prendersi cura di...
To run after	rincorrere
To take after	assomigliare/essere come...
Down	
To break down	rompersi/guastarsi
To sit down	sedersi
To slow down	rallentare
Over	
To get over	superare
To run over	investire
To turn over	voltarsi, voltare
Away	
To throw away	buttare via

FALSE FRIENDS

Actually	realmente, effettivamente	**Magazine**	rivista
Attualmente	**at present, now**	Magazzino	**warehouse**
Annoy (to)	disturbare, dar fastidio	**Novel**	romanzo
Annoiare, annoiarsi	**bore (to)**	Novella	short story
Annoyed	infastidito	**Occur (to)**	accadere
Annoiato	**bored**	Occorrere	**need (to)**
Comprehensive	esaudiente	**Phrase**	espressione, insieme di parole
Comprensivo	**understanding, inclusive** (di costi, servizi etc.)	Frase	**sentence**
Factory	fabbrica	**Realize (to)**	rendersi conto
Fattoria	**farm**	Realizzare	fulfil (to)/carry out (to)
Firm	ditta	**Sensible**	sensato, percettibile
Firma	**signature**	Sensibile	**sensitive**
Furniture	mobili	**Sympathetic**	comprensivo, partecipe
Fornitura	**supply**	Simpatico	**nice**
Library	biblioteca	**Synthetic**	sintetico (artificial)
Libreria	**bookcase**	Sintetico	**concise**

BRITISH ENGLISH VERSUS AMERICAN ENGLISH

British English	American English
Parole terminanti in *our* *Colour, favour, honour*	perdono la *u* *Color, favor, honor*
Parole terminanti in *tre* *Centre, theatre*	diventa *ter* *Center, theater*
Diversi passati irregolari *To learn, learnt, learnt* *To burn, burnt, burnt* *To dream, dreamt, dreamt*	 *To learn, learned, learned* *To burn, burned, burned* *To dream, dreamed, dreamed*
Verbi terminanti in *-ise* *Recognise*	*-ize* *Recognize*

USEFUL HINTS

HOW TO GIVE EXAMPLES

Example esempio

For example per esempio

For instance "

e.g. " (sempre prima dell'esempio)

We detected a variety of case, e.g. heart diseases that...

Such as come, ad esempio

Other departments, such as biotechnology...

HOW TO EMPHASIZE

To emphasize enfatizzare

To stress sottolineare, rimarcare

To point out far notare

To highlight evidenziare

To underline sottolineare

Remarkable notevole

Considerable notevole, considerevole

Impressive notevole, impressionante

Essential fondamentale, essenziale

Paramount assoluto, fondamentale

Of paramount importance.

HOW TO STATE CHANGES AND DEVELOPMENT

Development sviluppo

Trend, Tendency tendenza

To increase aumentare

To decrease diminuire

To improve migliorare

To deteriorate peggiorare

To enhance migliorare, accrescere

The report data showed a tendency in the use of prescription drugs.

The production of orphan drugs has been improved.

HOW TO EVALUATE

To evaluate valutare, stimare

To assess verificare, stimare

To estimate stimare

To overstimate/ to understimate sovra, sottostimare

Assessment valutazione

In our research, we assessed the efficacy of the drug.

The trial evaluated the side effects of...

AIM AND SUBJECT OF A STUDY

Aim scopo, obiettivo

To aim avere per scopo

The aim of this study is to evaluate the...

We aimed to evaluate...

Goal scopo, obiettivo

The goal of this study is...

Objective scopo, obiettivo

Our main objective was to determine whether...

Intent intenzione, proposito

The team's intent was to determine...

Purpose scopo, finalità

The purpose of this article is to...

To be intended to proporsi di, avere l'intento di

This study is intended to summarize...

To set out avere il proposito di

We set out to establish the safety of...

To attempt* cercare, tentare di

The team attempted to evaluate the risks of...

*slightly negative

To try cercare, provare

The team tried to evaluate...

Study studio, ricerca

They conducted a study on the effects...

The purpose of the study was to test the clinical...

Survey ricerca, indagine

A survey on orphan drugs was presented at the...

Review analisi, recensione

To review recensire, riesaminare

This review presents new evidence of...

The article reviewed the results...

Research ricerca, indagine

In our research we evaluated the potential...

In our research we assessed...

Report relazione, rapporto

The report illustrated the new system of...

Analysis analisi

The current analysis investigated the process of...

Essay saggio

In this essay we have tried to...

Work lavoro, opera

Our work examines...

Throughout this work we investigated...

Concern preoccupazione, interesse

Our concern was to state the value of...

In this analysis we concerned ourselves with the importance...

to concern oneself with sth. occuparsi di qualcosa

STUDY TYPE AND METHODS

Data* dati
All data are expressed as...
We obtained data about 2.000 patients with...
*verbo sia al singolare che al plurale

Questionnaire questionario
The questionnaire was designed for...

To query esprimere dubbi, indagare
Effectiveness was queried.

Rate of return/ response rate tasso di ritorno
The rate of return was.../The response rate was...

To record *registrare, annotare*
The registry recorded 10 operations on...

To monitor monitorare, controllare
Their aim was to monitor patients who...

Follow up proseguimento, che fa seguito a
On follow up at 2 years, some patients...
They planned to follow up the patients...

To follow up far seguito a

To collect data/ to gather information raccogliere informazioni
Data was collected for a new survey...
Our aim was to gather information about the...

AUDIO TRACKS